Fully Revised, Updated and Enlarged Edition

Homeopathy Cures where Allopathy Fails

Dr. S.C. Madan

M.B.B.S., F.R,C.S. (U.K.) M.N.C.H. (U.S.A.)
SENIOR E.N.T. CONSULTANT
HEAD OF E.N.T. TROMSO (NORWAY)
FORMERLY SENIOR E.N.T., CONSULTANT (U.K.)

PUSTAK MAHAL®

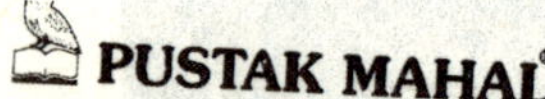

Administrative office and Sales Centre
J-3/16, Daryaganj, New Delhi-110002
☎ 011-23276539, 23272783, 23272784, 23260518
E-mail: info@pustakmahal.com
Website: www.pustakmahal.com

Branch Office
Bengaluru: ☎ 080-22234025, 40912845
E-mail: pustakmahalblr@gmail.com

ISBN 978-81-223-0725-2
Edition: 2026

Printed at : Sharma Printers, Delhi

Introduction

Dr. S.C. Madan holds M.B.B.S. from Punjab University, F.R.C.S. (E.N.T.) from Great Britain and membership in Homeopathy from U.S.A.

He has extensive experience in all branches of medicine, especially in his speciality of E.N.T. He was Chief of E.N.T. department in England and Scandinavian countries. He has been practising and teaching Ear, Nose and Throat for more than thirty years.

Dr. Madan has been using homeopathic medicines in addition to allopathy, from time to time, for the last twenty years, to help the sick in special situations where allopathy was bound to fail owing to its disastrous adverse effects or when it was going to give only temporary relief, compared to permanent cure with homeopathy.

Dr. Madan is convinced that homeopathy, if properly chosen, can give miraculous results in diseases like sinusitis, bronchial asthma, arthritis and gynae diseases, where allopathy is only palliative. He has brought to bear his extensive comparative knowledge of allopathy and homeopathy to the best advantage of the patient.

Dr. S.C. Madan
Mobile: 9958372312

Foreword-I

Dr. Subhash Madan is a well established experienced Senior E.N.T. surgeon in Delhi. He got his fellowship in E.N.T. from Royal College of Surgeons, Great Britain way back in sixties and practised there for some years.

On return to India, he has kept a full record of his patients here. He has observed through his own experience that the allopathic drugs have a lot of side-effects and in his majority of cases they do not benefit the patients to the extent he had thought them to. This made him shift his attention to the Homeopathy drugs. He went to U.S.A. to get training in Homeopathy. But that did not mean that he stopped surgery. He still believes and does surgery if it is needed. He is one of the top surgeons in his speciality in Delhi.

Going through the case sheets, he cites various cases where allopathic medicines have not worked and homeopathic medicines not only improved the condition of the patient but 'cured' their diseases. In a case of common cold, upper respiratory cattarrh or influenza, he has compared the allopathic cough syrups, anti-allergic drugs and anti-inflammatory drugs with the homeopathic drugs. In bronchial asthma, he seems to have cured even cases of status asthmatics. Similarly are the cases of diabetes and heart diseases cited.

These days with our vast scientific knowledge of various diseases, we allopaths try to find the real cause of the symptom which the patient presents to the doctor. The symptom, no doubt, is treated so that the patient gets comfortable, but these days more attention is paid to the cause or pathology of the cause of the symptom. In a case of common cold, URTI or flu, we modern allopaths prescribe cough syrups, anti-allergic drugs or anti-inflammatory drugs. All these drugs dry the throat and bronchial tree and, thus, produce more cough and bring in superadded bacterial infection. We give steam inhalation and if these are viral in origin, they get relieved within 3-5 days. If there is yellow or green sputum, we give antibiotics which have no parallel in homeopathic treatment. Similar are the cases of sinuses, throat and ear. Nobody, according to my knowledge, knows the cause of Bronchial asthma, but we know the precipitating causes and the pathology in the bronchi which produce asthma. We give relief to the patient by treating the pathological lesion of inflammation and constriction of bronchi but we cannot CURE asthma as we really do not know its cause. The World Health Organisation has researched on the medicines of Homeopathy and Ayurveda but none have been able to cure asthma. Similar is the case with diabetes, cancer and heart disease.

This does not mean that Homeopathy or Ayurveda systems of medicine are of no use. They are world recognised systems of medicine. They are cheap and side-effects are few. Allopathic medicines have great side-effects and are expensive. The side-effects have to be measured and weighed against the good effects produced by the drugs. Even Aspirin has a very bad side-effect of Haematemesis.

In the field of E.N.T., there are many chronic symptoms of nose blocking, sinusitis, ear and throat trouble, where at times even surgery does not help. According to Dr.

Madan, homeopathic medicines work wonders. Why not try and give these drugs to relieve the patients' misery. Similar should be the cases of other medical specialities. Moreover, I do hear from relatives, friends and some medical practitioners that for minor ailments, like headaches, pain anywhere especially in abdomen, loose stools where patients cannot wait and spend money for the test to find the cause of these symptoms, homeopathic medicines work and work well. But beware that you get the advice from a recognized homeopath like Dr. Madan who will give appropriate medicine and take less time to cure.

We, in medical profession, must have an open mind. Our sole aim is to give relief to the patient and to diagnose him properly. I wish Dr. Madan a great success in his sincere service to the mankind.

Dr. Prem Sobti
M.B.B.S. (Pb), F.R.C.P. (Ed), F.C.C.P. (U.S.A.), F.N.C.P. (Ind.)
President and Chief Physician, National Chest Institute and Research Centre, N. Delhi, Medical Adviser to WHO, SOUTHEAST ASIA

Foreword-II

For an optimum You, it is good news that you now savour Homeopathy. It is a servant's sangfroid version soaring high with eagle. Homeopathy aims at a permanent cure by removing the deficiency present in the constitution, which are mainly responsible for the various ailments. Once they are got rid of, health is restored permanently. The stipulation, however, is that it cures what is curable.

Homeopathy is not a catch-penny device to lure people in its fold. It is a veracious science though at times confusing and complicated but in the hands of a veteran a mighty weapon for cure. What is required is dedicated handling of the case.

A surgeon's total involvement and special interest in Homeopathy is rarely seen. Dr. Madan's practice of Homeopathy has brought him many laurels. His way of treating cases is very different. He understands that the primary obligation of a physician is to relieve the suffering and affect a cure, where the cure is possible.

Dr. Madan's stance is always research oriented. He is communicative and shares knowledge with others. His prescribing is spruce and steadfast. His book is a very good addition to the modern publications on the subject of homeopathy with very useful information, not elsewhere to be found. It is a very significant contribution to the subject which will provide new horizons to the profession.

Dr. Madan needs to be congratulated for this effort. Allopathy is generally condemned for its potent doses and crucial side-effects. Dr. Madan brings this torrent on a relative plane and successfully brings out the difference. The book should be counted among a marvel on Homeopathy.

Dr. Kulbhushan Bhardwaj
M.H.C., D.H.M.S., M.P.M.P.A., De.G.M., M.L.H.I. (Geneva)
Consultant Homeopathic Physician

Contents

Preface to the Third Edition

The contents of this edition differ from the first two editions in the following respects :

1. I have edited more complicated and more number of cases in it than in the previous editions.
2. The significant difference is that I have based my treatment not only on the principles of Hanemann, *i.e.*,
   a. **"Similar treats similar"**. Detailed history and symptoms are a must;
   b. **Aetiopathology;**
   c. **Mode of action of remedy;**
   d. **Combination therapy:**
   More often taking into consideration synergetic or antidotal effect of the remedies.

   Many of the homeopathic colleagues may criticise my this line of treatment but I have got the following reasons for using combination therapy.

   These days in high tech age, every patient wants quick relief. In view of the fact that many natural symptoms pertaining to a particular patient are masked by their taking drugs on their own or so many allopathic drugs already having been given before he comes to you, neither you nor the patient can wait for three or four consultations before you unravel the real symptoms.

The other reason for my using the combination therapy is that I have to select those combinations which are complementry to each other and their mode of action is identical and not antidotal.

Many times when the symptoms are very complex and do not fit into any constitutional remedy, then I have taken into consideration the underlying causative factors. These days by the time patient seeks specialist's advice, many allopathic and combination of homeopathic drugs have made a mess of the characteristic symptoms of the patient.

e. **Thorough examination of the patient:** It is a must as it is done in western countries by homeopaths.

f. **Modern diagnostic tools like CT, MRI, Ultrasound:**

However, like in the previous volumes where both allopathy and homeopathy had to be used where they are complementary, I have done so in this edition also.

In this edition, I have dealt much more complicated cases of gynae-obs. and nasobronchial allergy in infants and children, as it is becoming more and more common owing to increasing number of vaccinations and strong allopathic drugs used for various simple ailments. Two types of cases in gynae and obs., whom I have treated after they have had serious side-effects due to hormones, are:

1. Menopausal Syndrome.
2. Ammenorrhoea and Menorrhagia in young girls.
3. Prolonged lactation after weaning or scanty breast milk after delivery.

The other cases of advance vertigo, cervical spondylosis and sensineural deafness, Tinnitus and enuresis in children have also been given in this volume.

Sensarineural deafness is one ailment where there is absolutely no treatment anywhere in the world except giving hearing aid. Moreover, it is not within the scope of everyone's pocket to buy ear maskers.

In view of the tremendous stress and strain of modern life, both in students and sedentary life of business people, various new disease-entities have emerged which I have treated with homeopathy. Finally, in professional hazard diseases, in computer techs. and in persons working in call centres with air-conditioned surroundings, cases of cervical spondylosis and neuralgic pains are increasing at an alarming rate. After they had the 'quick-fix' treatment (allopathy) they come to me with symptoms of original disease still persisting **plus** the adverse effects of allopathy. Such complicated cases have been dealt with in details in this edition.

Vaccinations: A controversial chapter for homeopaths but is a booming industry for various pharmaceutical companies and for the paediatricians and general practitioners, I have clarified the facts and myths, advantages and disadvantages, remedies to counteract the side-effects of certain essential vaccines.

Finally, I express my sincere thanks to my son SOMESH, who worked very hard to compile, compute and rearrange various chapters in this third edition.

Finally, I express my sincere thanks to my wife Pamila, and my son Somesh, who were both responsible for encouraging me to write this book.

Preface to the First and Second Editions

This book is dedicated to the memory of my parents and brothers. In the last days of their ailment, I found allopathy had nothing much to offer except palliative treatment and prolonging their suffering.

My consciousness has compelled me to write this book in the best interest of the patient and to familiarize the medical practitioners (both Allopath and Homeopath) as to what is the best treatment for a particular ailment.

In my experience of more than 30 years, I feel disappointed to see the number of diseases caused by adverse and toxic side-effects of allopathic drugs.

Very often the disease created by allopathic drugs is worse than the disease for which the drug had been given. On the other hand, I have seen certain conditions which could be cured with a stroke of knife, but Homeopaths had been giving medicines for months and years, resulting only in the proving effects of the remedy and asking the patient in terminal stages to go to a surgeon.

My advice is while crossing the road, see both the Red and Green lights; only then we are safe. So is the case with medicine, whether allopathy or homeopathy.

We must compare the merits and demerits of a particular branch of medicine in relation to a particular ailment before implementing it.

Having had the experience of treating thousands of patients with allopathy & homeopathy and surgery, I can say with confidence that for most chronic diseases, allopathy is a failure and is only a smoke-screen against fire and does not remove the cause.

In acute conditions, allopathy, no doubt, acts as a miracle but to cure the cause, homeopathy is indispensable.

Comparison is the basic theme of this book. In brief, I have found homeopathy is safer, cheaper, curative and easily available. However, it cannot replace absolute surgical cases or life-saving antibiotics and there I have counteracted the side-effects of allopathic drugs with homeopathy, made the post- and pre-operative surgical treatment smoother and comfortable with homeopathy.

The purpose of this book is to bridge the gap between allopathy and homeopathy.

It will not be out of place to mention a few words about homeopathy which will be of help for an allopath to understand.

Homeopathy is essentially a natural healing process providing remedies to help the patient regain normal health by stimulating the body's natural forces of recovery. First connection between homeopathy and allopathy was small pox or DPT vaccination. In each case, a substance was taken in order to prevent illness.

VACCINATION is nothing but HOMEOPATHY.

LIKE TREATS LIKE is the basic theme in Homeopathy. Cold drinks can bring convulsions, if you take them when heated. Hot drinks can save you.

If a substance produces symptoms in a healthy person, the same person can treat a diseased person having the like symptoms, e.g., onions and garlic can cause sneezing, watery nose. These very substances can cure a person suffering from these symptoms. There is nothing strange about homeopathy, rather it has been an unrecognized part of our life.

Lastly, many homeopaths may be critical of my line of treatment as unconventional and not following the principle of Hanemann, by giving single remedy rather than polypharmacy (multiple). Things change, theories change with the changing circumstances. These days symptoms are complex owing to the use of multiple allopathic medicines. The other physicians may be critical of my using both branches of medicine (allopathy & homeopathy). My aim is to cure the patient in an economical way.

Homeopathy can act as a miracle, if applied correctly. Unlike the common view that homeopathy is absolutely safe, that is not the case. If used indiscriminately by quacks or for unlimited periods by amateurs, it can do more harm than good, as you will find illustrated examples in this book.

Finally, I discount the various theories and arguments put in various medical journals and in the media in Western countries, from time to time, that Homeopathy is not a science but Allopathy is a science. If that is the case, may I ask such advocates:

1. Was Thalidamide not scientifically proved before it struck its disaster?
2. What about Practolal (Eraldin) used in heart conditions in 60s which had to be withdrawn because of its side-effects. There is an endless list I can provide of diseases caused by so-called 'scientifically-proved' drugs. Recent examples are of Terfenadine and Cisapride?
3. Was Viox (Cox-B inhibitor) for arthritis not scientifically proved, before it is withdrawn suddenly?
4. Was Sysapride not scientifically proved, but now banned?

Conclusively, I would like to say that except in acute conditions or surgical conditions, allopathy should be used with caution, explaining to the patient the merits and demerits of the treatment.

It is a pity that in many states in U.S.A., Homeopathy is not allowed legally. I am of the opinion that those physicians who think Homeopathy is a farce, they do not know what they are missing.

I have the impression that if Homeopathy does not work, it is the homeopath who is at fault and not the Homeopathy.

In this book, I have dealt with (a) Common diseases; and (b) Intractable diseases.

I have given sample cases of each disease. Allopathic treatment has been given by other practitioners (specialists and general practitioners). Almost all cases after they have been dealt with by others, have come to me with not only the original disease untreated but also superadded diseases caused by allopathic drugs. They had non-disease miseries alongwith their principle disease.

I have given my line of treatment at the end of each case. I have also given common side-effects of allopathic treatment which the patients had when they came to me.

I found it essential to mention both types of treatments (allopathy & homeopathy) so that the patients know the green and red lights of their treatment and follow what is best for their constitution and ailment.

Lastly, I apologize to differ from the Homeopath colleagues of not going on symptoms alone and writing the book under various headlines of diagnoses. After all, diagnosis is based on signs, symptoms plus the modern diagnostic tools available. Symptoms constitute only part of the diagnosis.

If the patient is symptomfree in case of high blood pressure, or in certain tumours or in diabetes, does it mean he does not need treatment?

The last chapter deals with cautions and precautions in Allopathy and Homeopathy and diseases **caused** by doctors, unintentionally.

Two abbreviations used frequently are meant as: A.C.T. (Author's Comments and Treatments) and NSAID (Non-Steroidal Anti-Inflammatory Drugs).

Readers of this book might question me as to why I have not given potency and frequency of homeopathic treatment. The reason for such omission is "Homeopathy is tailor-made". Potency, doses and remedies depend upon the disease, symptoms, severity, resistance of the patients, previously taken medicines in homeopathy or allopathy. It cannot be generalized unlike Allopathy.

For convenience and safety, even a layman can take 30 potencies but other potencies and certain constitutional remedies should remain within the domain of a professionally qualified Homeopath.

Keeping in mind to CURE the patient safely rather than only treating and that also with side-effects, I have used Homeopathy, and at other times, Allopathy, and sometimes both, where they are complementary to each other.

Finally, I express my sincerest gratitude to three persons: My Guru and guide, Mr. A.P. Gulati, who initiated me into homeopathy, my wife Pamila, who has been the real force, and who initiated and pursuaded me to pen down my experiences, and spent sleepless nights to correct the manuscript.

Beyond doubt, the book would not have seen the light of the day without the efforts of the staff of Pustak Mahal.

1

Respiratory Diseases

COMMON COLD

Case I

Mrs. Sarita took decongestants for her upper respiratory infections.

Allopathy

Triominic, Action 500 and Vicks, all failed to give relief, then the doctor gave antibiotics, patient got better, but continued to have blocked nose, dry cough and wheeze.

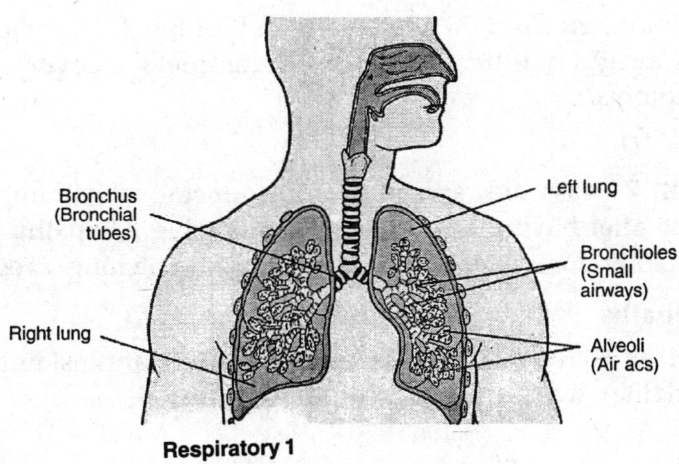

Respiratory 1

A.C.T. (Author's Comments & Treatment)

Effect of Allopathy

Blocked nose and ears, dry cough and wheezing, all due to drying effect of these decongestants.

Homeopathy

Antim Tart 30 alternate with Bell 30 + Phytolacca 30 and steam inhalation.

Case II

A child of 5 years with recurrent upper respiratory infections, thick yellow discharge from nose.

Allopathy

Sison (Antihistamine) Syrup with Amoxicilline, was given by G.P.

A.C.T.

Effect of Allopathy

Blocked nose, dry cough, irritability and loss of appetite. Blocked nose, dry cough was due to sison (Cetrizine) and loss of appetite due to amoxicilline.

Homeopathy

Antimonium Crud 30 alternate with Kali Bio 30. The child was alright within 3 days with complete recovery of symptoms.

Case III

Rohit, 7 years old, son of a family doctor, was brought to me after having been given the following Allopathy by his father for watery nose, sneezing and itching eyes.

Allopathy

Cetrizen Syrup for last six months. When antihistamine (cetrizine) was stopped, symptoms recurred.

A.C.T.

Effect of Allopathy

A child had a blocked nose due to dryness of nasal secretions caused by cetrizine. Drowsiness due to cetrizine, which affected his studies and normal alertness. The child, most of the time, was tired and lethargic.

Homeopathy

Arsenic alb 30 alternate with Gelsemium 30 both twice a day. At the end of treatment, Sulphur 30, two doses at 1-week interval.

Case IV

Gaurav, 5 years old, was brought with history of thick black, greenish nasal discharge coming in front and back of nose. He used to cough at night and vomit in the morning on getting up for the last two months.

Allopathy

General practitioners and ENT Surgeons had given him decongestants, cough syrup and antibiotics.

A.C.T.

Effect of Allopathy

Blocked nose, dry cough and wheeze, all due to decongestants and cough syrups.

Homeopathy

Pulsatilla 30 alternate with Kali Bio 30 and Bell 30 with steam inhalation.

The child was symptom-free, with good appetite in 3 days' time.

Most of the decongestants and cough syrups (allopathic) are simply a smoke screen against fire. These delay the treatment and do not remove the cause. By increasing

the viscosity and consistency of nasal and bronchial secretions, these simply increase the number of Sinus infections, Bronchial Asthmatics and Glue ears.

NOSE BLOCKING

It is one of the commonest and troublesome symptoms in infants and children.

Allopathy

Decongestant nose drops (Otrivin or Nasivion, Endrine).

A.C.T.

Effect of Allopathy

1. Temporarily relieves the blocking but after the effect of drops wears off, the blocking comes back.
2. Nose drops shrink the lining of nose temporarily and blocking is worse after the effect of drops wears off.
3. Nose drops are habit-forming.
4. Prolonged use causes Rhinitis Medica Mentosa (a disease of lining of nose).

Case I

A six-month-old baby was brought to me with restlessness and nose blocking which resulted after Bruffen was given for high fever.

A.C.T.

Homeopathy

Nux Vomica 30 – 2 doses at 1 hour's interval and steam inhalation.

For fever, I gave Aco. 30 + bell 6 + bry. 30 at 1-2 hours' interval.

Within 24 hours, fever and nose blocking disappeared like magic.

Case II

Four-year-old Rohit was brought to me for nose blocking and slight running of nose at times.

Allopathy

Cetrizine Syrup did not help.

A.C.T.

Homeopathy

Ammonium Carb 30, 3 doses at 1 hour's interval, cured both blocking and running nose.

Nose must be seen by an ENT surgeon before any medical treatment is given, since sometimes there can be a surgical cause for blocked nose.

TEETHING

Allopathy

Ibugesic (Bruffen) for pain due to teething and accompanying fever. Phenargen for running nose. Gramoneg (Nalidic acid) was given for loose motions associated with teething. Bruffen and Crocin were given for earache associated with teething.

A.C.T.

Effect of Allopathy

Stomachache was due to Bruffen. Dry nose and blocked nose due to antihistaminic. Glue ears were due to bruffen and antihistamine. They increased viscosity of the middle ear's secretions.

Homeopathy

Combination of Aconite 30 + Chamomilla 30 + Magnesium Phos 6x alongwith Biochem no. 21 act like magic minus the above side-effects of allopathic drugs. Sometimes, coffea 30, colocynth 6,30 are of tremendous benefit. This combination controls all the symptoms pertaining to teething.

COUGH AND COLD

One of the commonest ailments afflicting human beings all over the world. Mismanagement and **allopathic** treatment are the common causes of converting a simple cold and cough into chronic Bronchitis or Asthmatic Bronchitis.

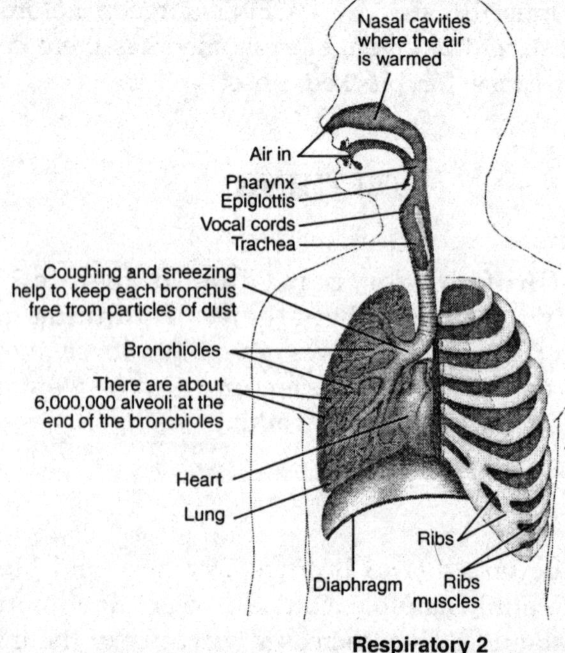

Respiratory 2

My following cases **exclude** cold and cough which are allergic in nature. These are dealt under **allergic Rhinitis and Bronchial asthma**.

There are four levels of severity of cold and cough and each level needs different treatment in Homeopathy.

A.C.T.

First Stage

This occurs on 2nd or 3rd day following cold and bad throat (often occurring as a result of junk food, e.g., chilled soft drinks, with preservatives, tomato sauce, laced food, spicy Chinese or Indian food).

Allopathy

Lozenges, Vicks, Decongestants like Actifed and Cough syrups with antiallergic as one of the ingredients and anti-inflammatory drugs like NSAID preparations (bruffen, ibugesic, flexon).

Effect of Allopathy

Dryness of respiratory tract secretions leading to heaviness of head and dry cough, excessive thirst and dryness of mouth. Anti-inflammatory and anti-histamine preparations lead to Sinusitis and Asthmatic Bronchitis by causing the respiratory tract secretions viscid and difficult to bring these out.

Homeopathy

Ipecac 30 alternate with Bell 30 + Phyto 30 with Kali Mur 6x + Ferum Phos 6x as complementary. Bryonia should not be given on the symptom of excessive thirst since excessive thirst is due to the side-effect of decongestants and anti-inflammatory drugs.

Second Stage

A.C.T.

At this stage, secretions are mucoid and easy flowing.

Allopathy

Decongestants (anti-histaminic and anti-inflammatory) along with Mucolytic agents (loosening the mucus).

Homeopathy

Arsenic alb 30 alternate with Bell 30 + Phyto 30. Giving such cough syrups (decongestants) is like putting kerosene and water (mucolytic agents) together in fire.

Third Stage

A.C.T.

There are thick, yellow, white secretions, sometimes easy and sometimes difficult to bring out.

Allopathy

Antibiotics with cough syrups. Antibiotics alone may work but **cough syrups** delay the recovery by causing the bronchial secretions becoming thick and viscid.

Homeopathy

Kali Bio 30 alternate with Ant. Crud 30 and Natrum sulph 12x.

Fourth Stage

A.C.T.

Most patients have come to me at this stage when the physicians have tried all the cough syrups, antibiotics and bronchodilators (opening of air passages). The following are record cases out of thousands which will demonstrate the ugly aspect of Allopathy. The clinical picture of patients coming at 4th stage after having all the antibiotics, cough syrups and bronchodilators, is that sinus throat and chest are affected at this stage. The following symptoms are caused by Allopathic drugs:

1. Oropharynx (inside of mouth) is parched and extremely dry. Patient says that the cough is dry but this cough is **false** dry due to the use of decongestants.
2. Patient is weak, tired and lethargic due to anti-histamines.
3. Patient is irritable due to the use of sympathomimetic (Triominic. actifed, dristan) preparations and Bronchodilators (deriphylline, asthalin).

4. Loss of appetite due to Gastritis.
5. Constipation and dry mouth due to use of antacids like Ranitidine.

"This is the gift of modern Allopathy for treatment of a simple case of U.R.I."

Homeopathy

Antim Tart 30 alternate with Merc Sol or Lachesis 30 gives dramatic improvement with steam inhalation. With my experience, Rumex, Spongia and Bryonia should NOT be given in such cases. **(Symptoms are modified due to allopathic drugs.)**

Case I

Archana (not real name) of 13 years, daughter of a renowned family doctor, was brought with intractable, apparently dry cough.

Allopathy

She had all the latest antibiotics including deworming medicines given by her father. No relief at all. Before coming to me, she was diagnosed by a chest physician who gave Augmentin and bronchodilators and decongestants. Physical examination revealed crepts at bases of lungs with thick-coated tongue and extreme weakness.

A.C.T.

Homeopathy

I gave Antim Tart 30, 3 doses at 2 hours' interval with Carbo veg 200 in the morning and at night. Kali mur 12x 4 pills in warm water TDS. Archana was O.K. in 72 hours.

Case II

A young lady doctor, 23 years of age, from Haryana, niece of a chest physician, was brought to me with history of cough and hoarseness for 2 months. All allopathic treatments had been exhausted without any relief. Antibiotics, Decongestants and Bronchodilators were of no avail. Physical examination showed Pharyngitis, Laryngitis and sub-acute Bronchitis.

A.C.T.

Homeopathy plus Surgery:

I suggested X-ray of sinus for which the patient told me that she already had 4 chest X-rays done during the last two months. These X-rays and blood tests were all normal. I insisted upon X-ray of Sinus which showed Mucosal thickening with fluid level. I did the Sinus puncture followed by Kali mur 30x – 4 pills TDS and Carbo veg 200 in the morning, Bell 200 at noon and Kali bio 200 at night. She was O.K. and went back to Haryana the next day after operation and phoned me to say, "I never realised the miracle of Homeopathy."

Advice: Chest physician must get X-ray of sinuses in a case of bronchitis, even with no symptoms of sinusitis, at the time of coming to the physician, since the patient forgets about having had sinus, after that has been treated with decongestants, long time back.

2

Ear, Nose and Throat

EXTERNAL EAR

Outer Ear: Fungus, Wax Accumulation and Otitis Extena (inflammation of outer ear)
It is due to bad habit of poking or cleaning the ear with cotton buds, towel, handkerchief or matchstick. If there is pain and swelling in addition to blocked feeling in the ear, it means superadded bacterial infection.

Allopathy

1. Antibiotics can control the bacterial infection but encourage the fungus formation.
2. Syringing is done to remove the wax.
3. For softening of wax, often Soliwax or Waxsolve ear drops are prescribed.

Effect of Allopathy

Because of turpentine in Soliwax, I have seen severe reactions. So is the case with dreadening allergic reaction to Chloromycetine ear drops. Syringing, unless done by an ENT surgeon, can rupture the membranes.

Homeopathy

1. It must be given only after cleaning the ear with Suction

Machine. After cleaning, I find Mulein oil is the safest and the best. Conium is rarely helpful.

2. Merc sol, bell, arnica, apis very often control inflammation.

MIDDLE EAR

Acute Otitis Media (Middle Ear Infection)

It is very common in infants and children as an accompaniment of teething or following U.R.I.

Allopathy

Often Phenargen Triominic, Sudafed, Actifed, Ibugesic, Tylenol Combiflam or Flexon are given along with antibiotics.

A.C.T.

Effect of Allopathy

Most of the subacute otitis media (Middle Ear Effusion) or glue ears are the by-products of the use of allopathic decongestants or NSAID drugs because of their tendency to increase the viscosity of secretions of nose and middle ear and stagnation thereby.

Homeopathy

Chamomilla 30, Belladona 6,30, Aconite 30 and Kali Mur 6x, 12x resolves majority of cases. Cases coming 4-5 days after the onset of ear infection respond to Puls 30, Bell 30.

Glue Ear (Middle Ear Effusion) or Subacute Otitis Media

I will describe this condition as a partially extinguished fire. As I mentioned earlier, it is a creation by allopaths because of the use of allopathic or anti-inflammatory drugs for a common cold or acute ear infection. Various decongestants and antihistaminics dry up the middle ear secretions accompanying a common cold, leading to middle ear effusion.

Allopathy

Myringotomy (opening in membrane) with insertion of Grommet (ventilating tubes): This procedure is done in epidemic proportions in western countries.

A.C.T.

Effect of Allopathy

The result of this surgical treatment is as follows:

1. Immediate improvement in hearing but condition recurs following another U.R.I.
2. Surgical hole becomes permanent perforation if infection supervenes.
3. Scarring at site of myringotomy.
4. It does not cure the basic cause, i.e., perpetual cold in a child – allergic or infectious.

Advice: In resistant cases of longstanding on decongestants, I do the myringotomy, but put the patient post-operatively on homeopathy to prevent recurrence of glue ears. After having used various types of grommets (T-tubes, Shah's etc.) for years, I am convinced that myringotomy, without putting the tube in, followed by homeopathy, is the best line of treatment.

Homeopathy

Lobel 30 or Merc Dulcis 6x, 30x, Borax 30 along with Kali Mur 6x often cures the condition.

I have seen cases coming from Homeopaths, being given Silicea and Kali Mur (dilutions). The Homeopaths had probably tried to bring out the secretions and, as a result, Silicea had led to perforation and Kali Mur (dilutions) increased the nasal secretions.

Chronic Otitis Media (Ch.O.M.)

Such cases are often of years standing with perforated T.M. and necrotic bone in mastoid with foul smelling discharge.

Allopathy

Surgical treatment is advised and done. The prime object is to save the life of patient because of threatening brain complications.

(Mastoidectomy or Tympanoplasty).

No guarantee that the ear would be dry, nor in every case, hearing is brought back to normal or even improved. The following cases will demonstrate the ugly aspect of failure of allopathic treatment.

A.C.T.

Case I

A child of 7 years suffering from discharging ear since the age of 3 years. There was no perforation but X-ray showed cholesteotoma. The child had a second opinion in U.S.A. and U.K. Everybody advised operation but nobody guaranteed that the ear will dry after operation. The child went to a nearby Homeopath who gave high potency of Silicea and Merc Sol. The child got worst ear discharge with blood-stained, foul smelling and scanty.

Homeopathy

I cured the patient in 2 weeks with Lapis alb 30 (on the principle of "like treats like"). It was blood stained discharge. The character of discharge made me prescribe lapis alb.

Case II

A young boy of 19 years was operated twice for Mastoid at a major hospital in Delhi.

Allopathy

Tympanoplasty (plastic surgery of ear) was done. He came with discharging ear. All antibiotics failed to cure him. Two operations for Mastoid failed to cure him. Examination showed granulations, and foul smelling discharge.

Homeopathy

After doing suction clearance, I applied Calendula Q + Thuja Q + Echinacea Q locally to the granulations. Internally, I gave Silicea 1M 1 dose daily for 3 days and this was followed by Calcarea Sulph 30 TDS for 2 weeks. His ear became absolutely dry. He had recurrence after 2 months which magically disappeared with Silicea 10M one dose only. I saw him after 6 months with no recurrence.

Case III

A U.N. official of 65 years had one Tympanoplasty done at Royal National E.N.T. Hospital at London and second in Geneva. 3 years after the operation in Geneva, he again got foul smelling, blood stained discharge in left ear and severe deafness. *Result:* Surgery and antibiotics failed to cure him.

A.C.T.

Homeopathy

Calcarea Iodid 30 alternate with Kali Sulph 30 both 2-3 hours a day. Ear dried up in 10 days. He was trouble-free for two years before he moved to U.K. and I have lost touch with him. Trying to close a medium or large perforation of T.M. with Homeopathy is wasting patient's and own time. However, Homeopathy does a wonderful job in drying up the ear before surgery.

Case IV

A 35-year-old lady with discharging ear (scanty, blood stained) of 5-6 years' duration, with complaint of leucorrhoea of many years, came from Kanpur.

Allopathy

Antibiotics, three times a day and various antifungal (local and internally) and antibiotics were used but without any relief.

A.C.T.

Effect of Allopathy

The above treatment failed to cure her ear or leucorrhoea.

Homeopathy

Hydrastasis 30 alternate with Kali Bio 30 and Biochem Kali Sulph 6x TDS cured the Sinusitis, Ottorhoea and Leucorrhoea. At the end of treatment, one dose of Thuja 200 was given since she had had vaccinations quite a number of times.

OTOSCLEROSIS

It is a disease of **Middle Ear** where Ossicles (small bones in Middle Ear) get fixed. As a result, mobility is restricted. The exact cause is not known.

Allopathy

Stapedectomy operation is ideal remedy, provided there are no contra-indications. Only in selected cases the results are good.

A.C.T.

Effect of Allopathy

1. Relapse occurs after some years.
2. Failure in some cases.
3. Hearing getting worst in other cases.

Homeopathy

Homeopathic treatment in the following cases will demonstrate the effectiveness of this treatment.

Case I

Husband of a lady doctor was operated twice at AIIMS in Delhi and after second operation hearing deteriorated to 70 db along with inner ear involvement.

Case II

A middle-aged lady had Stapedectomy (replacement of stapes bone in middle ear) in Lucknow, but 5 years after operation, with a bout of sneezing, the hearing dropped to 70 db. In view of failure of operation, she was not willing for operation. She also was a case of Otosclerosis.

Homeopathy

In both these cases of Otosclerosis, I gave Thiosinaman 200 OD and Ferrum Picric 6x TDS and hearing improved to 35 db.

INNER EAR

Meniere's Disease

A.C.T.

The symptoms of Tinnitus, deafness and, at times, Vertigo comprise the syndrome of Meniere's Disease.

Allopathy

Vertin, Serc, Stugeron, Stametil, Praxilene, Complamina, Tranquillisers.

In **intractable** cases:

1. Labrynthectomy and Shunt operations.
2. Tinnitus maskers.

Effect of Allopathy

In seventies, I did these operations in U.K. These operations cost enormously and surgical treatment has been extremely disappointing. Recently, I have treated advance cases of Meniere's Disease and syndrome from all walks of life with the following treatment:

More and more cases are coming these days because of prolonged and frequent use of Disprin for various

Cardiac and Neorological conditions and also NSAID preparations used for various anti-arthritic conditions.

Homeopathy

Acid Salicylic 30, Natrum Salicylic alb 30, 200, Causticum 30,200, Kali Phos 30. These Homeopathic remedies have magical results, provided these are used judiciously. These remedies have proved the old saying as correct: "To kill two birds with one stone." With most of these remedies, I have cured C. Spondylosis as well as Meniere's syndrome induced by NSAID preparations.

Case I

A.C.T.

Recently in 1997, during my assignment abroad, a lady of 48 years had been taking Atenolol (B-blockers) for High B.P. and HRT (hormone replacement) for menopausal symptoms, Proxilene for Meniere's syndrome, Ativan (tranquilliser) for anxiety and tension, but still feeling miserable and no improvement, whatsoever, in any of her symptoms. I suggested her Homeopathy. She laughed at first but when I reassured her and gave the following treatment she was 90% O.K. in 2-1/2 weeks when I left that country.

Homeopathy

Lachesis 30, Cimcifuga 30, Kali Phos 30. After a week's time, I increased the dose to Lachesis 200, Cimcifuga 200. The bases of my treatment for above symptoms are as below:

Lachesis: Primarily for High B.P. and menopausal symptoms.

Causticum 200: Controlled vertigo and tinnitus. Cimcifuga 200 controlled menopause and vertigo. Kali phos acted as a tranquilliser.

Case II

Mother of my receptionist had Meniere's Disease. She was 50 years old. All investigations were normal except some degree of perceptive hearing loss. She complained of severe Vertigo, loss of sleep and Tinnitus.

A.C.T.

Allopathy

Vertin, Alprax was given but did not give much relief.

Homeopathy

Natrum Salicylate 30 TDS was given for 1 week and she had 50% relief in all the symptoms in one week. Then I put her on Natrum Salicylate 200 once a day and in 8 weeks, she got completely cured. Biochem Kali mur was given in all the above cases of Meniere's Disease.

Meniere's Disease & Meniere's Syndrome

For a layperson, it will suffice to mention the symptoms of the above complex as:

1. vertigo. 2. noises in ears (tinnitus). 3. deafness.

In syndrome, it could be part of the above symptoms or all the symptoms.

My treatment in the following cases was done after investigations such as MRI andiometry (hearing tests) balance tests and X-ray cervical spine. All were normal but patient was still having very severe symptoms.

Allopathy

These patients who came to me, all had the treatment with stugeron, serc, stametil, rafecox — NSAID drugs and tranquillisers for tinnitus. Many had antidepressant drugs as well.

Homeopathy

Case 3. A very senior lady doctor, 65 years old, came to me after having been treated at Mumbai and Delhi by top-most neurologists, orthopaedic surgeons and psychiatrists.

She had severe vertigo, severe spondylosis, insomnia, depression. All investigations were normal, including MRI. Audiometry showed perceptive loss due to presbyacusis and due to prolonged use of NSAID drugs. X-ray of cervical spine showed some degenerative changes expected at that age. Examination of ears was normal.

Homeopathy

1. Conium and Lachesis at 200 potencies alternating with each other for 3 days had a magical effect and the doctor gained confidence in homeopathy and became hopeful of recovery.
2. Then I gave cocculus and cimcifuga and she was asked to discontinue all allopathic treatments. She was cheerful and happy for 2 weeks, when she again got relapse. She was having rapid pulse and high blood pressure (180/100). Her ECG was normal. She had been put on tenormin and alprax by an allopath doctor.

I gradually stopped tenormin and put her on tabacum, spigelia and cactus. The pulse became normal but high blood pressure still persisted. Then I gave aurum met and ignatia because of her depression as well. Her blood pressure came to normal.

Now she is managing without collar, sleeping without tranquillizers and no vertigo and no nausea. She is not taking any more stugeron or serc.

SINUSES

Sinuses are empty spaces in the bones of skull, normally filled with air. Inflammation of Sinuses with excessive formation of secretions from its linings, which may get infected is called sinusitis. It may be allergic in origin or infective or both. Sometimes bad teeth is the cause of sinusitis. In other cases, cancer could be the cause.

A.C.T.

Acute Sinusitis:

It often follows Common Cold, Viral Cold, Allergic Cold.

Allopathy

Decongestants (Actifed, Vicks Action 500, Dristan), Antihistamines (Claridine, Loridine, Cetrizine, Allegra) Anti-inflammatory drugs (Bruffen, Voveran, Ibugesic, Combiflam), Antibiotics are often given by allopaths.

A.C.T.

Effect of Allopathy

As far as my experience goes, Decongestants, anti-inflammatory drugs and anti-histamines have two roles to play.

Firstly, these are simply an eyewash and mask the symptoms without treating the cause. Secondly, these increase the viscosity of nasal and respiratory tract secretions leading to stagnation and blockage of ostium of Sinuses and **causing** sinusitis and not treating Sinuses. Thirdly, Antibiotics simply kill the bacteria without drainage of sinuses. Fourthly, Anti-inflammatory drugs simply relieve the pain and do not drain. These mask the true symptoms of the disease.

Homeopathy

Kali Bio 30 alternate with Bell 30, 2-3 times a day. If there is deviation of Nasal septum, it should be dealt with surgically.

Chronic Sinusitis:

A.C.T.

It is misconception in the patient's mind that nose blocking is a MUST symptom in a case of Sinusitis. It is not always true. Patient of Sinusitis presents with symptoms of complications of sinusitis. These usually present as below:

1. Earache
2. Asthmatic Bronchitis
3. Repeated bad throat
4. Bad taste
5. Bad smell
6. Frontal headache
7. Rheumatism
8. Chronic Eczema
9. Tired and lethargic feeling
10. Early morning nausea
11. Hoarseness of voice
12. Orbital cellulitis (inflammation of eye ball) Mismanagement of acute Sinusitis leads to Chronic Sinusitis. Bad dental hygiene is another common cause of Chronic Sinusitis.

Allopathy

Antibiotics, Decongestants and Antihistamines (Actifed, Terfendine, Bruffen) are often given by allopaths.

Effect of Allopathy

Complete failure to cure with allopathic medicines. Moreover, there are long-term complications due to Allopathic drugs. **Surgery** followed by homeopathic treatment gives a lasting cure.

Homeopathy

In the complicated cases, the following treatment can be advised:

Kali Bio 200 nocte, Calcarea Sulph 30 +
Belladona 30, 2-3 times a day.
In **advanced** cases, Pulsatilla 30,200.

For permanent cure intercurrent remedy is that Thuja 200, Silicea 200, 1M should be given.

Surgery and Homeopathy

In advaned cases, sinus drainage or cald-wel luc, followed by Homeopathic treatment.

SINUSITIS WITH BRONCHIAL ASTHMA

Case I

An experienced homeopath doctor, aged 30 years, came to me with history of severe headache, sneezing, nose blocking, premature greying of hair, letharginess, tired feeling and from time to time, urinary infection (told me on my questioning). These symptoms were for the last fifteen years.

Previous treatment

She had only homeopathic treatment with very occasional antibiotics when extreme. She had homeopathic treatment from her renowned teachers in Bangalore and in Delhi when her husband was transferred to Delhi. She had a very short spell of relief (2 weeks) in Delhi but again with severe symptoms.

The most distressing thing was that nobody had advised her a simple X-ray of sinuses, leaving aside CT scan.

I had the X-ray sinuses done, and there was marked fluid level in both sinuses with thick mucosal thickening, indicating chronic sinus with acute exacerbation from time to time.

All her symptoms (as mentioned above, including urinary) can be explained on the basis of sinus infection (any focus of infection in the body can cause recurrent urinary infection).

I advised her operation to sinuses. She refused initially but then after one week, she came crying with pain. After two days of treatment, I operated upon her when thick pus aspirated from both sinuses. She was very cheerful the next day.

However, to prevent recurrences of sinus infection, I had put her on Calcarea sulph and Kali sulph for a long time.

Reason

One should realize that at times surgery and homeopathy are complementary and not antidotal to each other. And moreover they cannot always dispense one with another.

I have seen Cal. sulph and Kali sulph very useful only **after** drainage of any septic focus is done. Without proper drainage these two preparations prolong the case.

For her chest and nose allergy which could be due to infecting organism of sinuses, I kept her on ars. alb and thuja. However, it is difficult to bring back black colour to her hair. Her headache, no doubt, has disappeared for which she was given spigelia, sangunaria and kalibio by her homeopath teachers, without any relief.

TONSILLITIS

Very often, when patients having repeated bad throat, with complications, like joint pains or ear complications or repeated missing of schools are advised operation to tonsils, they are reluctant to get operated. They think tonsils are supposed to protect the body, not realising that in their cases, unhealthy tonsils are adversely affecting their health rather than providing any protection. These unhealthy tonsils are spreading poison in the body. I have observed beyond doubt that unhealthy tonsils affect the height of children.

A.C.T.

This is one of the commonest diseases afflicting children more than adults all over the world. In India, incidence used to be less until recently with the junk food (Toffee, Raffles, Crisps, Chilled drinks with preservatives, Chewing gum, Tomato Sauce, Chilli Sauce, 'Gol Gappas') becoming more and more popular, incidence of tonsillitis is increasing. Prevention is better than cure. In Europe, kissing is one of the commonest causes of sore throat, if either of the partners is suffering from it.

Allopathy

Antibiotics is only a temporary relief apart from side-effects. **Surgery** in advanced cases is advisable.

Homeopathy

Can be divided in three stages depending upon the severity of Tonsillitis.

Early stage: Within 48 hours Bell 30 + Phytolacca 30 alternate with Biochem No. 10.

Middle stage: 48 hours after onset of Tonsillitis. Tonsils red with enlarged neck glands. Merc I.R. + Merc I. flav + Bell 30 alternate with Biochem No. 10. Sometimes Baryta Carb 30, 4-6 hours has to be added to it.

Late stage: There is a white pus deposit like Pseudodiptheric membrane and neck glands are enlarged. Lachesis 30, Merc Cor 30, Bell 30. For restlessness Aconite 30 can be given.

Caution: I have seen cases having been spoiled by the use of Hepar Sulph and Silicea with potencies absolutely irrelevant to the stage of the disease. Various patent preparations available in the market are many a times not suitable to the stage of disease and taken without professional advice, simply spoiling the case.

PHARYNGITIS

This is one of the commonest problems facing all over the world. Some of its causes are common to all patients irrespective of age or race or weather or religion rituals.

However, there are other causes which, in my experience after practising in different parts of the world and being in the speciality of E.N.T., are specific to certain habits of a particular community, harsh weather in certain countries.

A. Common Causes

1. Dental or Gum Infections

These are the common causes and often missed. There are very few people who use the tongue cleaners. Even I have seen some dentists who do not use tongue cleaners themselves though advising to their patients. The same way E.N.T. surgeons advise patients not to smoke and they smoke themselves (though not all). I strongly believe: "Practise before you preach." The deposits on the tongue are a good source of culture media for bacteria to grow than the other way round.

2. Sinus Infection

This can lead to chronic pharyngitis. One should not forget that sinus infection can happen from bad upper teeth apart from cold.

3. Gastric Acidity

Reflux in hyperacidic cases, whatever may be the cause of increased acidity.

B. Specific Causes

1. Eating or chewing irritating things in Asian countries are the common causes.

a. Tobacco chewing or Paan Masala.

b. Chillies, whether these are red or green. (Black pepper is irritant to the anus.)

c. Pollution, which again is more in Asian countries than in the west, is the cause of pharyngitis.

d. Smoky atmosphere in western pubs, crowded discos with hardly any ventilation for practical purposes again is the common cause of pharyngitis.

e. Kissing is another common cause of contracting pharyngitis, if the other partner is suffering from throat or gum infection.

f. Central heating in Western countries leads to dryness of the throat and leads to painful swallowing.

g. Allergic pharyngitis, especially due to 'dhoopbatti' and incense sticks burnt as religious ritual in certain communities.

h. Perfume sprays especially with strong odours.

I am stunned to see the number of cases of tonsil operations being done unnecessarily especially if they are willing to get it done privately, while these patients continue to have sore throat after operation since these are the cases who actually had pharyngitis and not tonsillitis.

From the foregoing paragraphs it is evident to take precautions accordingly rather than getting the disease and then having all the antibiotics and pain killers.

Treatment

Allopathy

It is very important to remove the cause after examination and investigation.

The common treatment is antibiotics and NSAID preparations like Bruffen, Diclofenac or Voveran. The side-effects of these are often stomach upset or repeated courses leading to piles, flatulence and skin allergies.

Homeopathy

Combination A.

I often give Bell + Phytolacca + Bryonia in 30 potency in acute cases. In chronic cases, I give only Bell and Phytolacca 200 potencies.

Biochem No. 10 is given as a complementary.

Case I

A 50-year-old lady came to me six weeks after the onset of sore throat, on having had homeopathic treatment, which caused increase in size of cervical gland and deterioration in health further with pain in neck, radiating to shoulder for which she consulted an Orthopaedic Surgeon who, after carrying out all investigations, excluded C. spondylosis and then she was referred to Maxillofacial Dental Surgeon who, after having done dental treatment with no relief, referred to me. On my detailed enquiries I came to know that Silicea 10M was given by Homeopath at the very onset of Tonsillitis. **Very high potency of Silicea at early stage of Tonsillitis had spoiled the case.**

Homeopathy

I gave this patient Merc I.R. alb + Merc flav. + Bell and Calcarea Phos 30.

GLOBUS HYSTERICUS

A.C.T.

It is one of the commonest ailments affecting 70% of menopausal and post-menopausal women in Western Europe. Patients complain of 'something in throat' and are afraid that this may be Cancer. This phobia about cancer leads to the following problems:

1. The anxiety about Cancer leads to stiffness of the muscles of neck, which leads to further increase in the symptoms. So a vicious circle sets in.
2. The reason for this symptom occurring at this stage is dryness of mucous membrane due to decrease in Oestrogen hormone just as in the case of dryness of vagina at this age.
3. Cervical Spondylitis and NSAID preparations taken for C. spondylosis are also the causes. Furthermore NSAID preparations cause further dryness.This leads to Globus Hystericus. In India, the commonest cause is indiscriminate use of NSAID preparations for any pain, leading to this condition.
4. Anti-hypertensive drugs lead to dryness of mucous membrane due to its drying effect.

Allopathy

Tranquillisers like Ativan, Alzolam, to allay the anxiety.

In India, anti-inflammatory drugs and antibiotics are given very often as a line of treatment by allopaths.

Effect of Allopathy

These allopathic drugs act as a smoke screen without removing the cause. Most of these tranquillisers are habit-forming. These preparations make the bread and butter of Gastroenterologist and Dermatologist by causing gastritis and allergic skin rashes respectively.

Case I

A.C.T.

A 43-year-old lady came to me at Batra Hospital a few years ago with the statement, "I have tried everything, every doctor, every hospital for the last 7 years without any relief to a feeling of lump in the throat." I asked her if she is taking anything for any other ailment of the body. She replied in the negative. On my cross questioning, she said, "Of course, I am taking various pain killers, but those are for my backache, not for the throat." The pity is that the backache still persisted.

In these days of superspeciality, specialists treat the patient fragmatically as if other parts of the body do not belong to the patient. Specialists, these days, treat (not cure) one part of the body belonging to their speciality and do not care of the adverse effects of their treatment on other parts of the body, thereby creating a disease for the other speciality.

Homeopathy

Coming to the above case, I stopped all allopathic pain killers. I advised saline gargles and plenty of fluids. The Globus Hystericus disappeared. However, I had to treat her backache with Homeopathy. For most cases, my treatment for Globus Hystericus is:

1. Reassurance that there is nothing sinister with the ailment.

2. Kali Phos 30 + Mag Phos 30, Avena Q + Alfa Q (after meals), Gelsemium 200 at night.

Case II

An Austrian lady, 50 years old, whose husband was posted in Delhi, had this problem of Globus Hystericus for 15 years. She had allergic throat also complaining of itching in throat near the palate (allergy to dust). She was put on Wyethia 30, 3 times a day, Gelsemium 200 at night. She had a dramatic recovery in two weeks.

HOARSENESS

There are numerous causes for the hoarseness. I will mention the common causes and then a few cases treated with homeopathy based on the **causation of hoarseness** rather than the symptoms which were similar in nature.

Firstly, after investigating them by Nasopharyngoscopy to exclude malignancy as the cause especially in smokers or at a vulnerable age of malignancy.

Having excluded malignancy as the cause, then according to symptoms, re-inforced by clinical examination, I have treated these cases:

Viral or U.R.I. (Acute)

Case I

A.C.T.

My wife's friend phoned in panic that her 3½-year-old child had suddenly become hoarse and asked me to advise on the phone treatment for her child which I declined to do so. Anyhow, she brought the child to my clinic.

Allopathy

The child was given Triominic and then Benadryl syrup for cold and blocked nose after Triominic failed to stop the cold by her Paediatrician.

Effect of Allopathy

After Triominic and Benadryl, voice became hoarse and child developed dry cough which was not before the Decongestants. Before she came to me, the mother took homeopathic medicine from a nearby Homeopath who gave Bryonia 30 on the symptom of excessive thirst and dry cough. In my opinion, these symptoms (dry cough and hoarseness) are due to Benadryl and Triominic given by allopaths.

Homeopathy

Carbo veg 30 alternate with Antim tart 30, both 2-3 hours a day. The child was O.K. in every aspect within 48 hours.

Emotional (Functional) Hoarseness

Sudden death news or fear can cause hoarseness.

Allopathy

Alzolam, alprax or ativan or calmpose are a standard treatment by allopaths for such cases.

A.C.T.

Effect of Allopathy

It is habit forming and acts as smokescreen without removing the cause.

Homeopathy

Gelsemium 200 alternate with Aconite 200 along with Kali Phos 6x.

Junk Food Hoarseness

A.C.T.

Spicy food (red and green chillies, tomato and chilli sauce, chilled soft drinks with preservatives, toffees, chewing gum, crisps, raffles) make the bread and butter of the doctor. These types of food cause inflammation of upper air passages due to inflammation of food pipe in surroundings.

Allopathy

Antibiotics and anti-inflammatory (Combiflam, Flexon etc.) given by the allopaths are often the culprit in increasing the hoarseness further.

Effect of Allopathy

The hoarseness persists although pain subsides. However, dry cough and gastritis result from allopathic treatment. Ranitidine is given for gastritis by allopath which further increases the hoarseness because of its drying effect on saliva.

Homeopathy

Bellis Pere 30, Bell 30, Capsicum 30, Citric acid 6.

Traumatic Hoarseness

A young lady came to me from Trans-Yamuna area in Delhi with sudden loss of voice after she shouted at her child.

Allopathy

The doctor gave her Bruffen.

Effect of Allopathy

The hoarseness had gone worse after Bruffen and thirst became excessive. Nearby Homeopath gave Bryonia on the symptom of excessive thirst not realising that it was drug-induced thirst.

A.C.T.

Homeopathy

On my examination, (Indirect laryngoscopy) it was found to be haematoma on the V. Cord. Three doses of Arnica 200 at 2 hours' interval followed by Rhus tox 200, one dose daily for 3 days, settled the problem.

Chronic Hoarseness

The underlying cause of chronicity must be found and dealt with such as smoking, drinking, spicy food. SINUSES and

Larynx must be examined to exclude Cancer or any other tumour. Excessive use or misuse of voice by teachers, singers, speakers, lecturers, clergymen can cause vocal nodules etc. in most of these cases.

Allopathy

Surgical removal of V. nodules by E.N.T. surgeons.

Effect of Allopathy

Hardly any treatment. Nodules often recur. Sometimes the voice is worse than what was before operation.

A.C.T.

Homeopathy

Voice rest. Arnica 200, Rhus tox 200 and Kali Mur 30 treatment to the causative factors.

Case I

A school principal from Nainital came to me with extreme hoarseness (could hardly speak) saying that she was better **before** two operations done to her vocal chords at two reputed hospitals of India.

Examination revealed that she was a case of marked Nasobronchial allergy with sinusitis and laryngitis. She was put on steroids and anti-histaminics by those E.N.T. Surgens..

Effect of Allopathy

The patient could hardly speak, after having had two operations, and lot of anti-histaminics.

Homeopathy

Without much hope, I put the patient on the following treatment, and to my amazement, she could talk to me from Dehradun in a very clear voice within a few days. The remedies were: Causticum 10M once a month.
Calcarea carb 200 once a fortnight.
Rest of the days: Kalibio 200 and Bell 200, once daily.

Case II

A very interesting case, typically the creation of illness by allopaths. A missionary sister, 50 years old, teacher by profession, was sent to me by a physician after she had treatment by two E.N.T. surgeons, one at Bihar and another at Kolkata for a simple case of upper respiratory infection.

Allopathy

The first E.N.T. surgeon in Bihar gave her Voveran-D (Diclofenac plus pseudoephedrine). The nose stopped running but the voice became hoarse.

The second E.N.T. surgeon at Kolkata teaching hospital, gave her antihistamine (Allegra-180 mg daily) for 3 weeks. The result was, she became completely aphonic, and had to strain her vocal cords before she could utter a word. The E.N.T. surgeon at Kolkata made the diagnosis of Reinke's oedema of vocal cords on indirect laryngoscopy and advised microlaryngoscopy.

A.C.T.

On my examination of the patient, the throat was absolutely parchment due to adverse effect of the treatment by the E.N.T. surgeons. The adverse effects are: Dryness by decongestants and anti-inflammatory drugs. Vocal cords were simply congested and failed to meet in midline owing to strain on their underlying ligaments without proper lubrication. The lubrication was taken away by voveran, decongestant and antihistaminics.

Homeopathy

Reasons for the following combinations:

1. I gave her Causticum 1M single dose. Causticum was given on the basis of weakness of cords (failing to meet in midline).
2. Combination of Ruta, Arnica was given on the basis of strain on the ligaments of vocal cords.
3. Carbo-veg for painless hoarseness associated with acidity owing to allopathic treatments.

The next day she calls me up saying, "What magic I have played!" Her voice had come back as a matter of fact soon after taking that 'puree' (Causticum) at my clinic, before she even reached home and took other combinations of mine. However, four days after my treament, she was absolutely fine. On her next visit, she brought another convent sister with similar complaint and following similar treatment by another E.N.T. surgeon and a general physician.

Unusual Case of Hoarseness

Case III

A 53-year-old male from Bangalore came with history of hoarseness for last 3-4 years. He had the laryngoscopy done there and the finding was that the right vocal cord was congested and there was paresis of left vocal cord. He was also seen by the neurologist who excluded any mediastinum growth occupying lesion as the cause of left recurrent laryngeal nerve paresis. It was presumed to be idiopathic as far as left vocal cord was concerned. He was given decongestants, antihistaminics by the surgeon, but the voice got worst rather than better. He went to Mangeshkar Hospital in Pune where after laryngoscopy and videoscopy, which impressed the patient immensely, the findings were the same as at Bangalore. They gave twenty pages of voice instructions to the patient, which did not make any difference.

In between he had homeopathic treatment by India's topmost homeopath of Kolkata who gave Hepar sulph which did not make any difference.

A.C.T.

Homeopathy

With efforts, I explored his past history and he told me that he had been having frequent severe headache for the last 4-5 years for which he had X-ray sinuses and there was evidence of advance sinusitis for which he was given antihistaminics and decongestants which worsened his hoarseness.

REASONS for the following combinations:

I first treated his sinus by surgery and then gave him **mucolytic and drainage** medicines followed by the homeopathic medicines as below:

1. Causticum and Carbo-veg because of left vocal cord paresis and acidity of stomach respectively.
2. Arnica and Ruta because of strain on vocal cords due to excessive and loud speaking.

He improved more than 50% in one week's time and then I advised higher and higher potencies to keep taking, going back to Bangalore. I have to get the feedback from him at the time of writing this book.

Conclusion:

I treated this patient on the following principles:

1. Chronic **infection** of sinus leading to congestion of vocal cord. I did sinus operation followed by antibiotic and drainage drugs.
2. **Misuse and overuse of voice:** Arnica and Ruta because vocal cord is ligamentous in structure.
3. **Paresis** of left vocal cord with causticum.

Case IV

17-year-old girl, Miss D, came with severe hoarseness for the last three years. She had been investigated at two top hospitals in Delhi and during her vacation in Kolkata, by Kolkata E.N.T. surgeons and top homeopaths.

In Delhi, she was also treated by homeopath after she refused operation as advised by E.N.T. surgeons, that they will do stripping of the vocal cords.

On my examination, she had multiple factors to account for her hoarseness:

a) She used to talk a lot.
b) She used to take lot of chillies and spices and chilled drinks.
c) She had chronic gastritis.
d) I noticed no emotional element in her.

Allopathy

The allopaths one after the other had given her decogestants and anti-inflammatory drugs like sudafed, bruffen and antihistaminics like cetrizine.

A.C.T.

In my opinion, these allopathic drugs have made the condition worst by causing dryness and increasing the viscosity of saliva. It is the most common and deplorable treatment for hoarseness I have seen not only here but abroad also, where still stronger decongestants are used for hoarseness.

Homeopathy

Reasons:

My line of treatment in this girl was as below, although it took three months to cure her, since bad habits of taking chilled drinks and too much talking are not easy to give up.

1. I gave Arnica and Ruta on the lines of excessive talking and strain to the vocal cords.
2. I gave Carboveg, Iris vers. and Acid sulph on the lines of increased acidity, and gastritis.
3. I gave her Capsicum on the lines of taking excessive chillies.

She was 90% better at the time of my leaving for abroad.

3

Allergic Diseases

A.C.T.

Hay Fever, Allergic Rhinitis, Bronchial Asthma, Eczema, Nasal Polypi are very common diseases all over the world and they are caused by pollution, industrialisation and use of stronger allopathic drugs.

Recently, St. Thomas Hospital in London gave the statistics as to how much the cost of treatment to asthmatic patients is going to increase in years ahead in view of anticipated increase in Bronchial asthma cases.

IMPORTANT FACTS REGARDING BRONCHIAL ASTHMA
(In Author's opinion)

A.C.T.

Firstly: I assert with confidence that there is **no** permanent treatment for Bronchial asthma in **allopathy**. All the modern nebulisers pale into insignificance compared to the properly selected homeopathic remedies.

Secondly: Some cases of bronchial asthma are hereditary but that is correct in 30% of cases only; the remaining 70% are due to acquired factors (junk food containing preservatives, environmental factors, more and more vaccination, side-effects of allopathic drugs, chronic infective focus in teeth, nose and throat).

Thirdly: Patients keen to have homeopathic treatment for bronchial asthma should realise that the road to successful cure is not straight and one or two consultations in chronic cases, especially those who had been on allopathic treatment, are not sufficient. Obstacles come during the progress of treatment which are dealt accordingly by changing the potency or the remedy or giving antiblock treatment, but cure is sure.

Finally: The longer the patient has been on allopathic treatment for any allergic conditions (Eczema, Migraine, Hay Fever), the longer it will take to cure asthma.

Out of 1500 cases of bronchial asthma I have treated, I will only mention a few specimen cases from my records of status asthmatic patients.

Firstly, I will deal with cases of asthma of **infants and children** since their treatment differs from that of adults as far as Homeopathy is concerned.

Case I

A six months' old baby, under the treatment of an allopathic Paediatrician, was one of my cured patients. Duration of illness was three months.

Allopathy

The baby was on deriphyllin, antibiotics, ventolin and parents were told to buy a nebuliser.

Effect of Allopathy

Baby still continued to have wheeze and was also irritable with loss of appetite.

A.C.T.

Homeopathy

Ipec 6 alternate with Bell 6, Biochem (NS 6x + KM 3x + MP 3x), Chamomilla 30 was given for irritability and teething. Within 24 hours, changes reflected in the baby.

Baby had a sound sleep, first time since the onset of illness. I continued the treatment for 3 more days when the baby was 90% better. Then I gave Thuja since in most children asthma is due to vaccinations. The baby was completely cured in one month's time.

Case II

A 7-year-old child was referred to me by a Paediatrician and the child was in status asthmatics.

Allopathy

The child was on nebuliser, steroids, deriphyllin. His physical examination revealed as very apprehensive, restless, nervous, cynosed with wheeze which you could hear from a distance despite all the above treatments. Nose and throat examination was insignificant.

A.C.T.

Homeopathy

Phosphorus 30(m), Bell 30 + Ipec 6(n) twice during the day. Arsenic alb 30 at night. Within 48 hours, the child was O.K. Phosphorus 200, 1 dose was given after 4 days. No other medicine that day. Next 4 days Bell 30 alternate with Ipec 30, 2-3 times a day. Two weeks after the above treatment, I gave Thuja 200, which is to be repeated every two weeks (four such doses).

Case III

A 3½-year-old girl. History of allergic Bronchitis since the age of 6 months, accompanying or preceded by bad throat or U.R.I. She had changed 3 Paediatricians since her birth. Basically, the treatments of all the Paediatricians have been revolving around the same medicine.

Allopathy

Triominic, Actifed Syrup, Ibugesic. For skin rash, Betnovate cream was advised to her.

Effect of Allopathy

Examination revealed irritable, fretful loss of appetite, glue ear (fluid in ear) but parents did not know about his deafness for two reasons: (i) They spoke loudly in the house; and (ii) Being given Ibugesic for fever, no complaint of pain either.

A.C.T.

Homeopathy

Antim Tart 30, alternate with Nat Sulph 30 twice during the day. Arsenic alb. 200 at night. 5 days after this treatment when the child was 90% better, Thuja 200 (once a fortnight) alternating with Calcarea Carb 200 (once a fortnight) was prescribed. The child was completely cured, when the mother brought the child for earache and six months later, the child had no attack of bronchial asthma, after the last treatment.

Case IV

A young lady, educated, widely travelled, and doing business, was suffering from status asthmatics. She was allergic to dust and could not tolerate any smell.

Allopathy

Even the nebulisers, steroids did not help her. She was given Tranquilliser to calm her nerves, but that too did not help her much.

A.C.T.

Homeopathy

Dramatic improvement with Ipec 200 in the morning, Moschus 200 in the evening and Belladona 200 at night. After 3 days, Phosphorus 200, Carbo Veg 30 + Lyco 30 (evening). Passiflora at night. Now, she is a family friend and I know she did not have any attack for the last two years.

Case V

An adult, fair complexion, plump man was referred to me at Batra Hospital by chest physician because of bronchial asthma, to exclude any E.N.T. as the cause of bronchial asthma.

Allopathy

Broad spectrum antibiotic, Bronchodilators and Steroids were given by allopaths.

Effect of Allopathy

Abdominal discomfort, disturbed sleep and still having the wheeze.

Homeopathy

On my advice to the patient that he should try Homeopathy, he scoffed at the idea saying, "When so many expensive medicines in allopathy did not do any good, how those small pills could work". Clinically, he had chronic Bil. maxillary Sinusitis and asthmatic bronchitis. No gastric problem. Occasionally he gets Eczema.

Nat Sulph 200 (M), Bell 200 (N) and Kali Bio 200 (N). In 5 days, patient was 70% better. Then I gave Medorrhanium 200 (once in fortnight) alternating with Calcarea Carb 200 (once in fortnight).

He was so happy to recover that he brought battalion of patients of different diseases from his neighbourhood to me.

Homeopathy treatment is not the same for two apparently alike patients. Self-treatment with Homeopathy for bronchial asthma is dangerous.

BRONCHIAL ASTHMA & SINUS

Case VI

28-year-old, thin fair lady, married daughter of a renowned and respected homeopath and sister-in law of a well-known allopath, came with history of 10 years of eczema, sneezing and bronchial asthma.

She had been most of the time on homeopathy by her father except during the acute attacks, her brother-in-law gave her allopathic treatment including steroids. In the past history, before marriage she used to have "migrain" attacks. Whether it was due to sinusitis or migrain, it is difficult to say in retrospect. She had only one sinus X-ray 5 years prior coming to me which was no doubt indicated sinus infection, but as often the case, she was put on antiallergic medicines but was not operated upon.

A.C.T.

Homeopathy, Allopathy & Surgery:

After getting a new X-ray, I strongly advised operation under antibiotic cover followed by homeopathy to prevent recurrence of sinuses and to treat her bronchial asthma with homeopathy. The father was reluctant for her to undergo operation. I strongly emphasised, NOTHING LESS THAN THAT.

Surgery

I operated on both sinuses, there was thick pus in both sinuses. She had tremendous relief in her headache ("migrain"—according to her). She was kept on antibiotics for one week followed by the following homeopathic treatment.

Homeopathy

1. I gave her Calc. sulph and Kali sulph to prevent recurrences of sinus.
2. I gave her Phosphorus and Arsenic alb for her naso-bronchial allergy.
3. Infrequently, I had to give her Thuja because of the supressions she had undergone with steroids.

It took two months to put this patient on the right track.

Conclusion

I must emphasise that sometimes another branch of medicine is a **must**, keeping in view the welfare, cure and safety of the patient. One should keep eyes open rather than having prejudices and aversion to other branches of medicine.

Case VII

One-year-old infant daughter of parents who are both allopathic doctors, got frustrated and extremely distressed because of their child repeatedly getting in and out of the Apollo and Holy Family hospitals in Delhi because of severe bronchial asthma.

Allopathy

Every two weeks the boy had to be put on intravenous steroids apart from steroid nebulisers. The grandfather of the child being a homeopath, suggested homeopathic treatment. They reluctantly came to consult for that since they did not have much faith in homeopathy.

The history goes back since the child was two weeks old, child was advised medicated shampoo for dry scales on the scalp. Since that time, the child has been suffering from severe form of eczema and bronchial asthma.

Homeopathy

I started treatment with Thuja 200, on the basis of having had BCG vaccination. The cough got worst, which I controlled with Arsenic alb and Natrum sulph 30 each alternating with each other. It came under control to almost 50%. Sometimes, sneezing, sometimes cough and running nose.

Before the parents came to me, they were given one dose of a certain homeopathic medicine by a top doctor in Delhi. They say the child skin allergy got worst. They do not know the name of the medicine. Since then, they were equally scared to have homeopathy as well.

Then I switched to Tuberclinum 200 one dose, followed by biochem no. 2 and 6 alternating with each other. I also gave combination of Chamomilla + Belladonna + Ipecac – all 6 potency, the child was 90% fit for 3 weeks, when one day again, he came with severe attack of asthma. On my repeated enquiry, this attack got triggered by "good night" used for repelling mosquitoes. So, then I gave Arsenic alb 30 alternating with Pothoes 30. The child has recovered almost 90%.

A month after that, the child again came with severe itching. Then I put him on Thuja alternating with Kali arsenic. Now the child has been fit for the last 4 months, and did not need any bronchodilators or steroids since then.

Case VIII

An 18-month-old boy, very hyperactive, extremely irritable, very restless, suffering from asthma since the age of six months. He was teething as well, also having severe bottom itching.

Allopathy

The child has been on usual treatment at various hospitals in Delhi, i.e. bronchodilators, nebulisers and steroids, both by intravenous and by nebulisers.

Homeopathy

After giving a dose of Thuja 200, I had given the following treatment:

Chamomilla, Coffea, Colocynth. He got very much better both in irritability and asthma, but continued to have bottom itching. Then I gave two doses of Cina 200 at the interval of 12 hours. The child was completely different, quiet as well as no attack of asthma until three months after that he came again with running nose and slight cough. Then I gave one dose of Tuberclinum 200 followed by throat medicine (combination of belladonna and merc preparation) since he was also frequently having congested throat, due to putting the finger in his mouth.

Now for the last six months, he is fine and with no complaints. He has been put on a maintenance dose of Biochem no. 2 and 6 alternating with each other.

NASAL ALLERGY

A.C.T.

This is one of the commonest ailments afflicting 75% of population all over the world. In Western Europe, despite cleanliness, due to greenery, high pollen content in the atmosphere is the cause of Hay Fever (pollen allergy). In the Asian countries (India, Bangladesh and Pakistan) dust and pollution make the bread and butter of medical professionals.

The other common cause of allergic Rhinitis being underestimated is 'Dhoop Batti' burnt by Hindu religious people.

Finally, herbal perfumes are equally responsible for allergy. House dust mite present mostly in carpets, curtains and airconditioned rooms is another common cause of allergic Rhinitis and Bronchial Asthma.

Allopathy

Antihistamines (Actifed, Terfendine, Stemiz, Cetrizine, Dimotap, Sudafed, Allegra) are the commonest treatment.

1. Longstanding cases with complications like enlarged turbinates, Steroid sprays or systemic use of Steroid.
2. If there is superadded infection, then antibiotics.
3. In big institutions like AIIMS and Patel Chest in Delhi, series of allergy tests are carried out and then desensitisation with increased doses of specific vaccine prepared.

A.C.T.

Results of Allopathic treatment are most depressing and disappointing in the field of Allergy as detailed below:

Antihistamines for allergic Rhinitis simply cause dryness and increase the viscosity of nasal secretions leading to Sinusitis and Bronchial asthma because bronchial secretions also become more viscid, thus causing narrowing of bronchioles, poor exchange of oxygen leading to respiratory distress. It is interesting to note some of the practical experiences of patients on **allopathic** treatment for their nasal or chest allergies as given below:

1. Patients, who had the allergy tests done at AIIMS or Patel Chest and found to be allergic to dust and H.D.M. or pollens, were advised to avoid dust and pollens.
2. Is this the practical advice? That means the patient should stop living in India or near greenery.
3. Some patients say that they were advised to block their noses with filters. Do the doctors know how uncomfortable these filters are? This itself initiates the attack of asthma.
4. Regarding desensitisation many patients go into aggravation of attacks of asthma or some cases go into anaphylactic shock. 15 years ago, I used to prescribe desensitisation vaccine from Beecham (U.K.). Good results in most cases were found but they had stopped manufacturing this vaccine for reasons best known to them.

Homeopathy

After using the allopathic diagnostic tool of testing for allergy, **I desensitise specifically with dilutions of Homeopathic preparations**. The dilution and frequency are decided depending upon severity of the disease in the patient and concomitant medicines the patient is having. In **non-specific** allergic cases of Rhinitis, I prescribe Ars alb 30, Natrum Mur 30, Gelsemium 30.

In **violent** cases of Rhinorrhoea, Ars Iodide 30.

For permanent cure at the end of acute stage, Calcarea Carb 200 (once in a fortnight) alternating with Sulphur

200 (once in a fortnight). These preparations are the domain of a professional Homeopath.

SKIN ALLERGY

Definition

Various names have been given to this allergy depending upon the cause. **Eczema** is the common name.

Common causes of Eczema (Allergic Dermatitis):

1. Due to increase in the use of strong **detergents**, strong **cosmetics**, tight, almost **airtight jeans and shoes**, nylon socks and nylon clothes make the ideal culture for the growth of bacteria and fungus.
2. People taking food with lot of **preservatives are prone to get skin allergy**.
3. Married Indian women using 'Sindur' in the middle of the forehead develop allergic reaction at that spot leading to falling of hair.
4. Strong medicated perfumed shampoos are often the cause of allergic skin reaction.
5. One forgets that dry skin is very prone to infection. If the normal lubrication of skin is taken away by **'After Shave'** lotions, which often contain high content of alcohol or spirit, one is sure to get skin allergy.

Following cases will give the insight of Allopathic treatment for skin allergies. **These allopathic treatments** are not only palliative but by their suppressive nature, these treatments are the *causes* of *Bronchial asthma, tumors, sciatica* and *paralysis*. Before I knew Homeopathy, I used to scoff at the idea of suppression. Now I have hoards of cases on record and I had cured by beating the suppression by bringing back the skin rash and then treating the skin allergy with Homeopathy.

Case I

A doctor practising in U.S.A. came to me with severe

weeping Eczema of legs, ankles, with thick gluey discharge. He is having this problem since infancy. Being from a rich family, he had been treated by renowned Dermatologists all over the world who had advised Antihistamines or Steroids, which, in India, even a quack can suggest. Patch tests done by Dermatologists revealed a few Allergens but hardly of any practical benefit to the patient. This doctor also had multiple Lipomas and Bronchial asthma.

Result

Bronchial asthma, Eczema, multiple Lipomas (recurring after removal), all were resistant to all allopathic treatments.

A.C.T.

Homeopathy

Natrum Sulph 30 alternate with Ars alb 30 and Hepar Sulph 3x, 2-3 times a day, for one week. Then after 7 days, Medorrhanium 200, 1 dose and next week Natrum Sulph 200 (M) and Petroleum 200 (N) Baryta Carb 200, Thuja 200, Conium 200 in cyclic order, each once in three weeks. In three months, he was 80% better. Finally, I gave Medorrhanium 1M one dose and he is cured and did not have relapse for nine months. But it is essential that he should avoid foods with preservatives, deodorants and antiperspirants.

Case II

An American lady, 45 years old, wife of a diplomat, stayed in different countries in Asia and had lot of vaccinations against any epidemic disease in that country, wherever she went. She suffered from severe Urticaria. She had taken latest antihistamines but as long as she took them she was O.K. However, soon on stoppage, Urticaria returned. She was sensible to refuse Steroids whenever the doctor advised.

A.C.T.

Homeopathy

Thuja 30 BD for 1 week. Then Thuja 200 once a week for

2 weeks, Urtica Urens Q TDS for 2 weeks. She was very much better but not completely. Then I did series of allergy skin tests and she was found to be allergic to house dust mite for which I gave increasing dilutions of **Homeopathic house dust mite** and she has recovered completely. She, then, brought her friend from Germany for treatment of allergic problems. This is an excellent example where I have exploited Allopathy and Homeopathy working in Unison. Diagnostic skin tests are done with Beechams Diagnostic test Kit. Desensitisation is done with Homeopathic Dilutions, which are safe and convenient.

Case III

Myself (Author) had itching eruptions (Papular) on the abdomen and forearm's inner surface 15 years ago. Dermatologists advised anti-allergic, ointments and cream, but I did not take any of these.

Homeopathy

I took Natrum Mur 1M which dramatically cured. I often take excess salts and that is why Natrum Mur 1M cured my condition.

Case IV

I developed weeping Eczema six years ago on the ring finger. I attributed to the use of Betadine for scrubbing before operation.

Homeopathy

Arsenic alb, Natrum Sulph and Petroleum failed to give relief. Finally, Thuja 30 BD cured. Reason for taking Thuja was that I had numerous vaccinations when going to different countries. The second reason for taking Thuja was that I had Sebaceous cysts on forehead. This disappeared when I took Thuja 200 once a week.

20 years ago, I had Sebaceous cysts and were removed surgically, but these recurred more voraciously a few weeks after surgery.

URTICARIA

Allopathy

I have treated 50 most resistant cases of Urticaria after they had systemic and local steroids until these patients had to stop these because of tremendous side-effects and relapses of the Urticaria.

Homeopathy

Urtica Urens and Apis 30, 200, 1M have given very good result. To give a permanent cure, I had given them Natrum Sulph 200 alternate with Thuja 200, once in fortnight in rotation. Other cases had permanent cure only when I gave Medorrhanium 1M fortnightly.

Case I

A middle-aged lady came with swelling of lips and nostrils. On my questioning, she admitted that she also had swelling of vulvovaginal opening.

Homeopathy

Acid nitric, 30,200 based on the fact that rash affected skin-mucous membrane junctions, gave dramatic results.

Case II

A teenaged girl was very fond of eating Chinese food, getting hives soon after eating, and she kept antihistaminic in her purse.

Homeopathy

Ant. crudum and Pulsatilla cured the patient in 2 days' time.

Case III

In non-specific cases, I often succeed with Rhus tox, Apis and Arsenic in 30 potencies.

Case IV

Recently, a young pregnant lady came with severe reaction

in the ear with chloromycetine ear drops as advised by her E.N.T. surgeon. She could not take any allopathic antiallergic medicine due to pregnancy, so I cured her with Homeopathy.

Homeopathy

Apis, Bell and Arsenic alb, 30.

Case V

Recently I got an interesting case. An Italian man based in Delhi developed itching rash while fishing on holiday in Canada. He came back and doctors in Skin Institute and AIIMS in Delhi treated him as infected eczema, and also put him on steroids, which he reluctantly accepted since as an educated well informed person, he knew the side-effects of steroids. After having all sorts of treatment and having developed the side-effects of treatment, he came to me with the original disease worse than when it started.

Homeopathy

I gave him Rhus tox. 30 four hourly and he got cured in three days' time.

4

Women Diseases

MENOPAUSE (Climatric)

Climatric Changes

This is a recognised entity these days than two decades earlier.

It occurs in both the sexes but the symptoms are more pronounced and more lasting in women than in men.

The severity and degree depend a lot on the pre-existing nature of the patient.

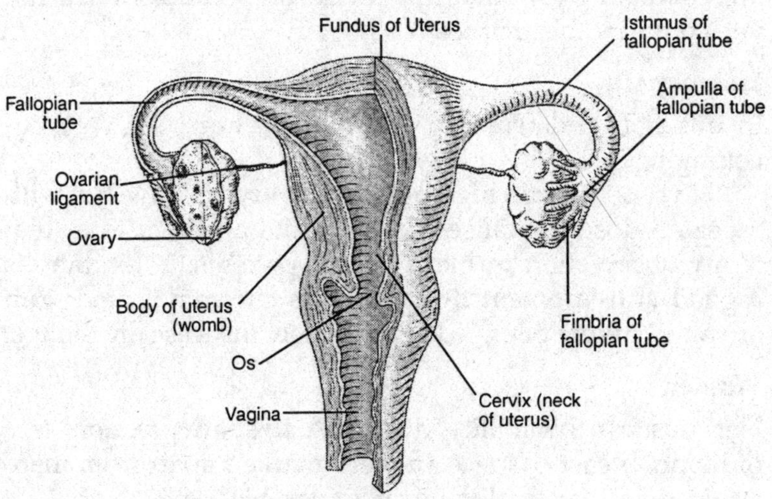

Female Reproductive System

This is considered to be due to hormonal changes in both the sexes.

It will be dealt with separately in both the sexes with comparative treatment of allopathy and homeopathy.

Men

Often the symptoms are reduced sexual libido, irritability and depression.

Allopathy

The treatments often given are testosteron and anabolic steroids. These preparations may give a feeling of exhalted mood and well being but one should not underestimate the susceptibility of prostate cancer with these preparations, and onset of diabetes and hypertense with steroids.

To increase the libido, though they may say that viagra has revolutionised it, agreed, but recent researches have shown that most elderly men who need viagra are also on nitrate preparations, and vasodilator effect gets potentiated which can be dangerous.

Though new advances have shown that central nervous stimulation drugs which lead to sexual arousal are comparatively safer, but these preparations have not yet come in the market.

Homeopathy

In this field, homeopathy has equally not been very encouraging.

Lycopodium in high potency is very effective but with repeated doses, it causes the opposite effect, at least that is my observation in many of my patients. Yohimbine is a good anti-impotent drug but it is contraindicated with anyone having piles, which is often the case in oldage.

Women

Nervousness, irritability, disturbed sleep, depression, loss of libido, breast changes are very marked apart from menstrual disturbances like very heavy bleeding.

Introspection of their emotions helps many of these women.

Allopathy

Recently, beyond doubt they have found that cancer of breast and stroke are more common in women who are put on these hormonal preparations than what it was thought earlier — the usual U-turn in the "research of allopathy".

Recently, it has been found that there is more mortality due to stroke and gastrointestinal bleeding *due to aspirin,* if aspirin taken for prophylactic who had no coronary or heart attack.

The conclusion is that aspirin should be given as a preventive who already had a coronary or heart attack and not in those who had no heart problem.

Homeopathy

If the correct remedy is selected, I have seen these act as a boon. I have given this subject in detail under different symptoms of menopause in women, such as high blood pressure, menorrhagia (excessive bleeding, loss of libido, depression, anger, facial hair and breast changes).

A.C.T.

This surprises many of my colleagues as to what made me prescribe Homeopathy in this speciality, while most of the time I am busy in Middle Ear Surgery.

A couple of cases given below will demonstrate as to how I could cure the nose and ear blocking of the patient only after stopping the Allopathic treatment for menopausal syndrome (H.R.T.) the patients were taking from Gynaecologists and Endocrinologists.

Case I

An educated lady coming from a doctor's family complained of nose blocking, heaviness of head, sensitive to noise.

Allopathy

She was taking H.R.T. by a top Endocrinologist of Delhi and at the same time, Lasix by a physician to overcome retention of water due to H.R.T.

Effect of Allopathy

On her first visit to me, she categorically said "No" to my advice of stopping the Hormone treatment, because she said that it has been advised by an Endocrinologist of international fame. He has told her that H.R.T. will stop the Osteoporosis and will prevent Coronary A. disease. He did not mention the dangers of Breast Cancer due to H.R.T. (Hormone Replacement Therapy). This woman had hysterectomy for Fibroids 5 years ago. Ovaries were not removed.

Homeopathy

She was very nervous, apprehensive and all the time on tranquillisers

Apis 30 (M), Cimcifuga 30 (D), Lachesis 30 (N). Passiflora Q, if she did not get sound sleep. She was 50% better in one week. Then I gave 20 potency of each of the above medication and she improved 70%. Finally, I gave Oxytropis 30 TDS and she was on top of the world. (The patient is of nervous temperament, trembling and tense.) So to cure her E.N.T. problem I was forced to treat the Gynae aspect of this case. She had no more nose blocking and stopped otrivine nose drops which she was having for years. As a result, I feel pity on the number of menopausal and post-menopausal aged ladies suffering more from side-effects of H.R.T. than due to menopause.

Allopathic treatment at times seems to be worse than the disease. Modern Patch treatment of hormones has not made much difference.

Menopause and Hormones

This is the most debatable subject all over the world till date. As often the case with most of the cases, so to say, scientifically proved, in allopathy, there is reversal of opinion now as regards giving hormone in menopausal syndrome. Until a couple of years ago, H.R.T. (Hormone Replacement Therapy) was considered to be a boon and was supposed to prevent osteoporosis and heart attack. Now recent researches show, as reported in the recent medical journal in Britain, that hundreds of British women are suing American drug companies for damages, because of suffering from strokes and cancer allegedly caused by H.R.T. It is now said that it increases the risk of breast cancer by 26% and strokes by 41% taking it for five years.

Case II

Homeopathy complementary to Allopathy:

An educated woman, 47 years old, suffering from menopausal symptoms (hot flushes, lethargininess, depression, rheumatism, irritability and putting on weight) had hysterectomy at the age of 32 years. Ovaries were not removed. She used to complain of severe left-sided headache and discharging right ear on and off, not responding to allopathic or homeopathic treatment for one year before she came to me. The problem of treating her allopathically was that she was allergic to most of allopathic treatments.

I treated her allopathically only under the umbrella of Homeopathy. I gave Sulphur 30 every morning and antibiotics for the ear. Sulphur controlled the allergy which could have occurred due to the antibiotics. The ear dried up completely for the first time. Somebody suggested that it is Sulphur rather than antibiotics which had controlled the ear infection, but that is not the case since she had Sulphur in different potencies from a Mumbai Homeopath without any relief.

For her menopausal symptoms, I gave her Sepia, Cimcifuga, Apis and Lachesis. To cure her depression, I gave her Aurum Met 200 alternate with Ignatia 200 once in a fortnight each.

DEPRESSION AT MENOPAUSE

It is again one of the common symptoms which expresses in a bizzare form. Many women say that they cannot describe their symptoms.

Depression exhibits in the following forms:

1. Sadness.
2. Loneliness.
3. Restlessness.
4. Heaviness of head.
5. Irritability.
6. Loss of interest in surroundings and everyday life activities.
7. Anxiety.
8. Sexual aversion.

Allopathy

1. Alprax, Calmpose, Larpose, and other antidepressants such as prozac—all of them have side-effects of causing dependency, habit forming, gastric upset and increase in weight.

2. The other treatment which allopaths give for menopausal depression is to put them on H.R.T. which has its own side-effects. Recent theories have established that stroke and breast cancer are more common in women who are taking harmones compared to those not taking them.

It is just the U-turn of various allopathic theories.

Homeopathy

1. I find Pulsatilla, Sepia, Ignatia and Kali phos are of unquestionable value.

Either singly or in combination, depending upon the symptom complex of the patient, especially her nature, are of unquestionable value in menopausal depression.

Reason for the above combination:

Changing mood and weeping tendency of pulsatilla.

Sexual aversion and "a fish out of water" attitude at menopause, with sagging of uterus, typical of sepia.

Irritability, depression and disturbed sleep, confused emotions of Kali phos.

The above combination has given me best results in my patients than given individually.

HOT FLUSHES AT MENOPAUSE

This is a common symptom in 90% of women at menopause. If the woman does not know at its first onset, she gets panicky as something serious is happening. It is worst in highly stung women due to instability of autonomic nervous system.

Allopathy

We do not have any treatment except to give her hormones, which have their own side-effects. Less than hormones some physicians give alprax to calm their nerves. However, alprax like other tranquillizers is habit forming and in the long-term may lead to Parkinsonism.

Homeopathy

1. Sangunaria and Glonoin is my mainstay in this symptom. It must be sang.candedis and not nitrica. We should start with 30 potency of Glonoin, then go to 200.

2. Those patients who did not respond to this, I gave them 30, 200 potency of Lachesis which often controls the symptoms.

3. In very resistant cases, and those who had migrain in the past, I gave them Sulphur 30, 200 at infrequent intervals, followed by Sangu. and Glonoin.

Reason for the above combination:

Sangu.can and Glonoin in combination has much better results owing to their synergestic action than given alone. I have found that **Lachesis, in combination with other remedies, has a negative effect.**

MENORRHAGIA AT MENOPAUSE

It is one of the commonest diseases and at times becomes a dire emergency. 45-year-old Mrs. M had vicarious bleeding lasting too long and too profuse.

Allopathy

She was treated by three gynae-obstetricians but got no relief with Dicynene, Gynae C.V.P. Capsules and Botropase. Ultrasound was normal. D & C done when the bleeding stopped, was normal. But she started bleeding again 2 weeks after the previous allopathic treatment and the Gynaecologist wanted to put her on H.R.T. but the patient refused. This time she was bleeding from nose in addition to P.V. bleeding.

Homeopathy

Trillium Q + Hammelis + Blumia Q (5 drops of each mixed together in a glass of water), 1/2 to 1 hourly depending upon the severity of bleeding. This is alternated with China 30. She is absolutely O.K. for the last two years. China controlled the weakness associated with bleeding apart from its action as a haemostat.

MENOPAUSE & RELIGIOUS INSANITY

At menopause in women, apart from nervousness, irritability, disturbed sleep, hot flushes, vaginitis, the other common symptom which I recently was confronted with three women, was insecurity which they replaced with extreme degree of religiousness which was almost on the verge of, I will say, insanity, because their rationality of mind was lost.

Allopathy

The allopaths had given these women tranquillizers (Ativan) and antidepressants (Prozac) which simply made them drowsy and lethargic and they started putting on weight, which further made them conscious of their figures and went further into depression.

Homeopathy

Case I

A lady of 48 years, whose husband was alcoholic, changed to Buddhism. Although believing in any religion is not right or wrong, but what made me think of her in terms of insanity is when she completely lost rationality of mind under the spell of religion of course such patients do not admit that they are under the spell of religious insanity.

Many women get inclined to spiritualism near menopause. As to which hormones are related to religious insanity, I have not been able to pinpoint.

Under the spell of religion, this lady started finding faults in everyday's life and in everybody's actions leading to the fact that she was viewing sex as a sin and according to her whosoever was having sex, will go to hell.

Their family life became a hell as her husband and grown up child and daughter-in-law told me.

I gave her sepia first as one of the menopause medicines, but that did not have much results. Then I put her on agnus and caladium as she also complained of vaginal itching, common at menopausal age.

In between these two remedies, I had to give her oxytropis because of her nervousness.

It took three months when she developed a rational attitude to life and religion.

The lesson in this case is that there was **REPLACEMENT OF INSECURITY WITH RELIGION**. Even the great psychologist Froid labelled extreme degree of such devotion is nothing but insanity.

VAGINITIS
(Vaginal Itching at Menopause)

This is often caused by dryness of vagina at menopause due to hormonal changes (low content of oestrogens).

Allopathy

Various vaginal creams (antibiotic and antifungal) with Metrondizole by mouth (Fasigyn).

A.C.T.

Effect of Allopathy

Apart from Gastritis due to metrondizole and anti-inflammatory drugs, at times there is severe local reaction to pessaries and antibiotics and hormonal creams. Itching recurs a few days after stopping the medication.

Homeopathy

Apis 30, 200 alternating with Acid Sulph 30 and Helon Q after meals. In resistant cases Thuja 30 followed by the above treatment. Ambra is an excellent remedy in vaginitis at menopause. In my experience, Caladium is not of much help.

EXCESSIVE URINATION AT MENOPAUSE (CYSTITIS)

This is one of the most intractable condition amongst women at this age.

Allopathy

Urologists and general practitioners keep giving antibiotics one after the other. The condition recurs again after you stop the antibiotics. One must realise that once the urine is sterile on culture and the symptoms are still persistent, then it is the irritable bladder which is causing frequency of urination, just like irritable bowel syndrome. But allopaths have nothing much to offer except asking for repeat cultures and changing antibiotics one after the other, the way they keep dosing with first generation of norfolx to fourth generation of floxacine in irritable bowel syndrome.

Homeopathy

My line of treatment in such cases is to treat on lines of irritable mucous membranes, whether of bladder, or colon, once the culture is negative. I hope the urologists will agree with me if they are not conscious of prestige issue of being an allopath.

Welfare of the patient and cure should be the prime aim of any treatment.

1. I often give Causticum, Cantharis, Mercurius and Passiflora. The potency of Causticum varies from patient to patient. One of my patients gave no response until I gave 10M of causticum at one month's interval.

Caution to Homeopath

It is very important to note that uterus prolapse is the cause of frequent urination due to pressure on the bladder. This cause must be excluded at this stage.

Case I

A British lady on holiday to India came to me through one of my treated patients asking for homeopathic treatment for her backache and cystitis.

A.C.T.

Allopathy

She has taken tons and tons of norflox and its sister antibiotics in U.K. but has been getting recurrences for the last 6 years. She has also been taking bruffen for her backache, lots of vitamins for her mouth ulcers and omeprazole for gastric reflux and acidity. She has also been taking metrogyl for her vaginal fungal infections and vaginal pessaries.

Here is a typical example of making a mess of patient's ailment by allopathic treatment, thereby causing uninvited non-disease miseries as explained below:

a. Mouth ulcers were due to bruffen and metrogyl
b. Acid reflux was due to bruffen and antibiotics
c. Vaginal fungal infection was due to side-effects of broad spectrum antibiotics for urinary infections:

Homeopathy

I gave her berberis-Q which controlled most of her urinary infection and backache. Then I gave combination of causticum and cantharis and merc. i. rubra.

She had no recurrences for the last three years.

Reasons for above remedies:

1. On the basis of cause.
2. On the basis of clinical examination.
3. On the basis of **knowledge of side-effects of allopathic drugs.**
4. On the basis of law of similarity.

Excessive urination is also associated with Vaginitis. Owing to proximity to vagina, there is irritation and due to short straight urethra in women, soon cystitis occurs. So there is vicious circle.

Vaginitis causes cystitis and cystitis causes vaginitis.

A.C.T.

Allopathy

Antibiotics control the bacterial infection but most Gynae-Obs. undermine the overgrowth of vaginal fungal infection because of the use of broad spectrum antibiotics for cystitis. May I ask the Urologists as to what explanation they have got after the urine is sterile in culture, but the patient still has frequency of micturition. Here Homeopathy has surpassed Allopathy.

Homeopathy

"Like treats like". Cantharis alternate with Berberis V. with Equisterum Q after meals has controlled the most obstinate cases of cystitis at menopause.

Homeopathy and Allopathy

In some cases, both have to be given where they are complementary to each other. The classical example is of cystitis with vaginitis alongwith backache. More than 50% women suffer from this ailment after menopause. My line of treatment in such cases is as below:

Allopathy

I give Lactobacil in the form of sporlac which looks after fungus of vagina.

Tight under clothes especially synthetics, tight jeans are the commonest source of growth of bacterial culture in the humid atmosphere. Hot Humid atmosphere at genital region makes the medium proper for bacterial and fungal growths leading to **Vulvovaginitis.**

Homeopathy

Locally: Mixture of mother tinctures of Hydrst. + Thuja + Calendula.

Internally: Apis 30 + kreosote 30 alternating with mixture of arn. 30 + nit. acid 30 + ambra 30.

If there is backache, then Berberis Q will act as boon. However, in suspected cases, Pap smear and Biopsy should be done to exclude any sinister condition before giving the above treatment.

SKIN RASHES AND ITCHING AT MENOPAUSE

Allopathy

The common treatment all over the world is one or the

other form of antihistaminics (cetrizine, clarytin, loratidine, avil, phenargen). If these rashes are not controlled by antihistaminics, then they give steroids.

The side-effects of antihistaminics are excessive dryness of nose and mouth and they may complain of nose blocking or painful throat despite there is no infection. The worst thing is that there is more dryness of vagina on its pre-existing dryness due to low oestrogens. That further leads to itching and excoriation of vulva.

Moreover by suppression action of antihistaminics, we push the underlying cause deep inwards which later on make its appearance in the form of tumours or sciatic pain.

I have already mentioned about the side-effects of steroids at various stages in my book.

Homeopathy

This treatment is tailor-made.

Case I

A 47-year-old lady came with intractable itching. Antihistaminics used to work previously, but not anymore. Now she was forced to take steroids.

I had put her on Natrum mur 1M single dose because of her chronic anxiety. She got 80% relief. Then I gave a dose of lachesis 1M. (She could not tolerate tight clothes and had slightly high blood pressure). Now it is six months since I gave this treatment and she has forgotten about the rash.

OSTEOPOROSIS AT MENOPAUSE

This, no doubt, is a big bugbear to most women at menopause.

Allopathy

In the Western countries, most women take calcium effervescent or with Antacid preparations since it has to be taken for a long period. They forget the adverse effect of calcium on kidney, especially in acidic medium since most women are fond of taking acidic things.

Homeopathy

Comparatively, Calc. phos 6x + Calc. fl. 6x 2 pills of each TDS for long periods are safer than allopathic calcium. (Shell cal.)

HYPERTENSION AT MENOPAUSE

It sets in many women at the age of menopause.

It is such a common entity that it is futile to put all women on antihypertensive drugs whose blood pressure goes up due to cetain mood swings or hormonal changes, unless the blood pressure is persistently high and other causes of hypertension are there.

A few cases mentioned below demonstrate that we should treat the underlying cause, which, in such cases, is hormonal imbalance.

Case I

Mrs L, 47 years old, came as an emergency case, with severe vertigo, nausea, heaviness of left side of chest. Things got aggravated when thinking about it to be a heart attack. The blood pressure was 190/100.

Allopathy

The cardiologist kept her under observation. ECG, Echo and lipid and other blood investigations were normal. Then he advised angiography, which the patient declined.

He put her on sorbitrate, disprin, stugeron and envas 5. Following was the reaction of this patient to this treatment:

a. Severe headache, which was due to sorbitrate, not going away with disprin.
b. Disprin caused severe constipation.

c. She got irritating cough due to envas which almost went into bronchospasm for which deriphylline had to be given, which caused palpitation and restlessness and loss of sleep apart from stomach upset.

Stugeron, no doubt, controlled her vertigo and nausea.

The patient refused to take any of these medicines and came under my treatment for homeopathy.

Homeopathy

1. I started the treatment Lachesis 1M, no other medicine that day.

   I gave Lachesis because my diagnosis was that her hypertension was **due to menopause**, after excluding all other causes. At the commencement of Lachesis, her BP was 200/105. The next day her blood pressure came to 160/95.
2. Then I followed three times a day Aurum met and Ignatia, knowing the nature of that woman. The blood pressure came to 140/90 after 3 days of treatment. She could have a sound sleep.
3. For her vertigo and nausea, I gave her Cocculus, that worked as a miracle and also controlled her fear as well.
4. Then I gave her Spigelia and Arnica, that controlled her left side chest pain, though ECG was normal.

Case II

A family friend, 46 years of age, was having severe Hypertension and other mild menopausal symptoms.

Allopathy

She was under treatment of an eminent Cardiologist who tried everything for her Hypertension, but she got adverse effects due to allopathic drugs. Her BP range was 240/120.

Homeopathy

Lachesis 200 at night with Passi Q + Rauwolfia + Crategus (1:1:1) after meals alternate with Baryta Mur 30 2-3 times a day. BP came to 130/80 but shot up again after a week. On my enquiry as to whether it was due to any emotional cause, she replied, "No". But her son told me she had recently strained relations with her daughters-in-law. Ignatia 30 alternate with Kali Phos 30 2-3 times a day brought the blood pressure down to 130/80.

Case III

A German lady, 48 years old, married to an Indian and settled in India for the last thirty years, came to me with the following symptoms:

Allopathy

She said she is a case of HBP (190/100) for which she is taking envas 5.

She has got high cholesterol and lipid for which she is being given statins.

She has got insomnia for which she is given alprax.

She has got gastric acidity for which she is being given ranitidine.

She gets hot flushes which she manages without H.R.T. and refused to take though prescribed by gynae.-obs. since she knew its side-effects through media.

She had extremely annoying and irritable cough for which she originally came to me to exclude any problem in throat. She had taken all sorts of cough syrups advised by her specialist.

INSOMNIA, DEPRESSION AT MENOPAUSE

Allopathy

Calmpose, Alzolam and Hypnotex, Alprax, Prozac are often given.

Effect of Allopathy

Habit forming and long-term use of these cause Parkinsonism and depression.

Homeopathy

Kali Phos + Coff + Gel + Valer in combination often give a sound refreshing sleep.

Recent Concepts on H.R.T.

Recent research at Wake Forest University Bapist Medical Center says:

They find no evidence that oestrogen supplements protect older women against heart disease. This information is sufficient to compel pre and post-menopausal women to think twice about their need for synthetic hormone replacement. Also consider the study of National Cancer Institute in U.S.A. which concluded that 8.6 million people are taking H.R.T.

According to Dr. Judyth R.Ullman and Robert Ullman, new studies at women taking combination of oestrogen and progesterone reveal that they are at significant higher risk of developing breast cancer (8% a year).

MENOPAUSE & SEXUAL DESIRES

Diminution of sexual desire, in some cases even aversion, is a common complaint, though not many women speak openly with this symptom in the Asian culture, unless you specially elucidate it. The usual phrase is that "I have gone off sex." Some go to the extent of hatredness as illustrated in the following case. Such women, who develop hatredness against the forces of nature, I have found them extremely nervous and settle for nothing less than Oxytropis and Ambra in homeopathy.

Case I

A 43-year-old lady came to me with a diagnosis of sinus headache. She also complained of nose blocking and X-ray sinuses showed mucosal thickening. So I operated upon her sinuses and put her on mucolytic drugs. She got only partial relief. Then I went to her marital history and she told me that since the cessation of her periods, she will be the last person "to allow her husband to come near her". She said that since she has become a Buddhist, she abhors sex, she has acquired supernatural powers. Here is a case of **menopausal sexual perversion, and gets delusions.**

Homeopathy

I gave her a dose of conium alternating with lachesis. That completely changed her life to happiness. It was like killing two birds with one stone. It controlled her high blood pressure also for which she was being given envas. The envas was causing intractable cough which also stopped once she did not need envas as her blood pressure came under control with conium and lachesis.

Case II

An allopathic lady doctor, 52 years old, came to me suffering from head to toe from all the diseases you can think of. In my opinion, more than 70% of her ailments were caused by allopathic medicines, which were available with her as she was a doctor.

Allopathy

She had the following symptoms and took the following allopathic medicines before she came to me:

1. Severe vertigo with spondylosis for which she had taken cox-b preparation and voveran, which had caused gastritis.
2. Gastritis, flatulence and haemorrhoids due to constipation which itself was due to omeprazole.
3. She had insomnia for which she was being given alprax.
4. Severe depression for which topmost psychiatrists of Delhi and Mumbai had put her on anti-depressants.
5. Finally, she had developed Parkinsonism. (In my opinion it occurs due to prolonged intake of tranquillizers and antidepressants — the "gift" of modern treatment by allopaths).

Homeopathy

I started her treatment with natrum mur 1M. The next day she phoned up to say she had a natural sleep for the first time in 10 years. As expected, after a few days, again she got depressed and hypochondriac with aversion to sex. I gave her Conium which acted like Electric Convulsive Therapy (E.C.T.) of allopathy completely bringing her old memories to the surface. Then I gave her some counselling and she was put on a maintenance dose of Ignatia and Aurum met and for her spondylosis and vertigo, Cocculus and Cimcifuga have done magic to her. Luckily, her husband has been very supportive who had extensive knowledge of psychology and I asked him to do counselling to her.

Reasons for giving above remedies:

1. Natrum mur is par excellence a remedy in chronic depression and mortification.
2. Conium works like Viagra in women, who have aversion to sex.
3. Cocculus and Cimcifuga work on the cerebrospinal complex and never fail me in cases of spondylosis and vertigo, its action based on aetiopathology.
4. Ignatia and Aurum met are based on the principle of "similar treats similar" and can be compared with prozac in allopathy.

CYSTITIS

Case

A Kashmiri girl, 23 years of age, had chronic U.T.I. She was unmarried. There were 30-40 pus cells and 8-10 R.B.C. in urine. Ultrasound of abdomen did not reveal any Calculus. Due to previous use of repeated antibiotics, her W.B.C. was 3000. She was extremely weak and not a suitable case to be put on antibiotics due to low W.B.C.

Homeopathy

I put her on Cantharis, Equisterium Q and Berberis V.Q. She was symptom-free in 1 week with normal urine report. For her debility, I put her on China and Acid Phos and she was back to college in one week.

LEUCORRHOEA

Case I

A 27-year-old girl had Leucorrhoea for 5 years. The discharge was acrid, and had great weakness and debility with constipation.

Allopathy

She had D&C and vaginal pessaries but the condition used to recur a few days after stopping the treatment.

Homeopathy

Alumina 30 alternating with Natrum Mur 30. She was O.K. in 3 weeks' time, both in leucorrhoea and constipation.

Case II

A 46-year-old lady was with yellow, greenish foul smelling leucorrhoea. Tiredness, debility, low blood pressure, weakness were associated symptoms.

Allopathy

Three times D&C with antifungal and antibiotics and hormonal vaginal creams she used, but had only temporary relief. Finally she took Nazral by mouth and she developed severe Thrombocytopenia and Leukopenia due to Nazral and blood transfusion had to be given.

Homeopathy

Sepia 30 alternate with Kali Bio 30 for 1st week, Kali Mur 6x TDS, Pul 30 alt with Borax 30 for 2nd week. She is O.K. and has no complaint since then.

Case III

Leucorrhoea in a little girl of 10 years with slimmy, curdlike white discharge, itching and redness at vaginal opening.

Allopathy

She was advised by gynae.-obs. antibiotics and antifungal creams but used to get only temporary relief.

Homeopathy

Calcarea Carb 30 alt. with Puls 30 both twice a day. Ovatestis 3x once a day cured her leucorrhoea.

Case IV

An old woman of 65 years, debilitating, case of burning itching of vagina, prostration, tired feeling, dragging down sensation of vagina with prolapsed uterus.

Allopathy

Prolapse operation was done but recurred after 18 months.

Homeopathy

Helonias 30 alternate with Sepia 30.

Case V

Wife of a foreign diplomat, 35 years of age, was one of my successfully treated patients. She had treatment in U.S.A., Canada during the time when her husband was stationed there and had taken the latest allopathic treatment but got no relief. She had **blood-stained, scanty foul smelling vaginal discharge**. She was not diabetic. D&C with Pap Smear ruled out any malignancy.

Homeopathy

Calcarea Iodid 30 alternate with **Lapis alb 6** with Thuja 200 once a week (2 doses). She got completely cured in seven days. She stayed in India over 18 months after my treatment and had no relapse.

AMENORRHOEA
(Absent or Scanty Periods)

This disease is of two types, e.g., **primary** and **secondary**. Primary is more difficult to treat. **The following case is of Primary Amenorrhoea.**

Case I

A 20-year-old girl was treated by a renowned Endocrinologist of India in Delhi for 3 years with various hormone preparations. She still did **not** get periods but she got Cushing's syndrome (moon face, unwanted hair on the face and breast), B. asthma, depression, insomnia and Osteoporosis as a **result of allopathic hormonal treatment.**

On examination, she had well developed secondary sexual characters but not the periods.

Homeopathy

I gave treatment to her in two stages:

Firstly: to treat the complications of allopathic treatment (mentioned above).

Secondly: homeopathic treatment for her Ammenorrhoea. For her depression, I gave Aurum met 200 in morning and Alfa Q + Ave Q after meals twice daily. For her cushing's syndrome, I gave Apis 30 and Apoc. Five Phos 4 pills, 3 times a day as a complimentary to the above regime. She took 3 months to recover from complications of allopathic treatment.

For Amenorrhoea I gave her Phosphorus 200 alternating with Lycopodium 200 for one week. She got the periods and got married, though did not have any issue.

Case II

A 23-year-old married lady from a village did not have periods at all. I asked my Gynae colleague to give me her finding in this case and she was found to have no uterus.

This case illustrates the importance of physical examination even in homeopathy.

Secondary Amenorrhoea is common, but often the result of frequent use of hormones leading to side-effects of hormones (facial hair and obesity) which lead to depression and inferiority complex.

Case III

Miss N, 22 years old, unmarried, had secondary Amenorrhoea for the last few years. Hormonal study and ultrasound were normal. This girl was sensible to refuse hormonal treatment as advised by gynae-obs. So the case was uncomplicated.

Homeopathy & Reason

She came under my treatment for Homeopathy. She was very emotional, weeping while narrating her story. I prescribed Aconite 30 alt. with Kali Phos 30 for 1 week and Pul 30, Sep 30 and Cim 30 in cyclic rotation. She got the periods.

SECONDARY AMENORRHOEA

Case IV

A young, very fair complexion allopathic lady doctor, 24 years old, came to me after having allopathic treatment for seconday amenorrhoea at topmost teaching hospitals in her state (U.P.) as well as in Delhi teaching institutions. She had many times hormonal assay tests done where prolactin level was somewhat higher. She was repeatedly treated with hormonal preparations with withdrawal bleeding.

Unfortunately, she was having side-effects of these hormones, e.g., increase in weight, leading to inferiority complex, irritability, disturbed sleep. If she stops the hormones, then she does not get periods.

A.C.T.

On my questioning, she told me that irregularity of periods started with her stress near board exams.

After seeing hundreds of such cases, I am of the opinion that hormonal disturbances start with some stress and strain which through the hypothalamus disturb the regularity of hormone secretions leading to amenorrhoea or menorrhagia.

It is a different thing in case of primary amenorrhoea.

The treatment given by gynae-obs. in such cases are tranquillizers and hormones. Anybody can imagine as to how a doctor can work under the influence of tranquillizers which this doctor patient was being given.

The steroid type side-effects of these hormonal preparations are well-documented (hump neck, facial hair, increase in weight).

Reasons for the following combinations:

Homeopathy

1. *Combination 1*:
   For stress and strain: Ignatia + Kali phos.
2. *Combination 2*:
   Pulsatilla, Cimcifuga and Apis. Apis was given because she developed polycystic ovaries due to these hormonal preparations. She had normal ovaries before these preparations were given. Although allopaths do not agree with my theory, Pulsatilla and Cimcifuga were given as these are the head remedies for regulation of menstrual cycle.
3. *Combination 3*:
   Senecio-Q + Gossipium-Q has given me splendid results in resistant cases.
4. *Combination 4*:
   For her Dysparunia (painful coitus), I gave caulophyllum + mag. phos + colo. + moschus). My this combination is excellent antispasmotic for vaginismus.

It took me two months to bring this patient to normality with smiling face, good sleep, less irritability.

Case V

A 30-year-old woman with two children came with the following symptoms: a. irregular periods for the last 18 months for which she has taken three courses of hormonal treatment from two different gynae-obs. She developed the following complications as a result of allopathic treatment:

a. Acne.
b. Increase in weight and facial hair.
c. As a result, there is marital discord, thereby unable to sleep without tranquillizers.
d. She has become hypersensitive fighting with her husband over trifles.

Homeopathy

Reasons:

I started with Thuja 1m owing to the fact that tetanus vaccinations are given as prophylactic during pregnancies which lead to bizzare symptoms. Then I followed with Gossipium and Senecio, both in mother tincture. Finally, I gave apis 200 twice daily.

As a result, her weight had come down, her hair growth receded but still the periods did not become regular. Then I gave one dose of Sulphur 200 and put her on Cimcifuga and Chamomilla, being a very highly irritable and, at times, depressed person. Then I put her on Ignatia and Aurum Met which killed two birds with one stone, controlling her blood pressure and irritability.

Case VI

A young girl of 23 years came with secondary amenorrhoea for the last four months. She had no other problems except that she used to get severe constipation on and off due to low fibre diet.

Homeopathy

I cured her amenorrhoea with high fibre diet and gave a combination of aesculus + collinsonia and alumina.

Conclusively, I will stress the point that it is very easy to treat secondary amenorrhoea (unless some gross hormonal abnormality). The treatment becomes difficult when they have already been treated with hormones.

MENORRHAGIA
(Excessive Vaginal Bleeding)

These cases are becoming more and more common since hormonal treatment for various gynae ailments cannot be properly monitored despite the sophisticated and expensive tests. As a result, these treatments overshoot the mark and lead to excessive bleeding.

Case I

Mrs. C, 38-year-old, a **very interesting case,** came to me with little hope of any cure with homeopathy but on the persuasion of her elder sister-in-law, whose menopausal bleeding I treated with homeopathy, she came to me. She was very dejected as she was told by renowned gynae-obs. of Delhi that hysterectomy is the only answer. On top of it, her one sister-in-law died recently because of cancer of uterus. Furthermore, her illiterate mother-in-law convinced her that she must get the uterus removed if she wants to save her life.

In Investigations:

D&C and biopsy ruled out malignancy. The ultrasound showed endometrosis. In the past, she used to get leucorrhoea for the last 10 years for which she had all the modern treatments and she got adverse side-effects such as menorrhagia and colitis with allopathy.

Now, I had to treat her for the following:
a. fear of cancer
b. overweight
c. facial hair
d. menorrhagia
e. endometrosis
f. leucorrhoea alternating with bleeding.
g. colitis.

Homeopathy

Reasons:

1. Phosphorus helped her overcome fear of cancer and control her bleeding.
2. Alumina and Borax were given to control her leucorrhoea. These two remedies were given because she was feeling very weak and had constipation also.
3 Five phos, was given as a complementary to the above remedies. This brought up her haemoglobin from 7 mgm to 10 mgm. She could not take allopathic iron since it would cause colitis on a pre-existing colitis which was due to metrogyl preparations given for colitis.

She is a different person now, very cheerful as the ultrasound has also shown 90% improvement compared to the previous ultrasound. There is no leucorrhoea, no weakness. She is now on a maintenance dose of cimcifuga, pulsatilla and sepia – all in 30 potencies.

Most of the remedies were given on the principle of Hannemann (similar treats similar). Nosodes were given in between like THUJA and CONIUM.

Case II

This is another interesting case of a lady doctor, 47 years of age, working with W.H.O., who was on official tour from USA to Colombo and she had to make an emergency halt at Delhi owing to severe vaginal bleeding. Her relatives in Delhi suggested homeopathic treatment which she reluctantly agreed upon after having two bad experiences in USA with allopathic treatment with no significant improvement apart from the side-effects of hormonal treatment.

After listening to her story and seeing the ultrasound, I told her that she has got menopausal bleeding. She became paranoid and furious on hearing the word 'menopausal'. She said that how could it be menopause when all the hormonal tests done in USA showed these are normal. As the human psychology goes, she still desired to be called a young girl since menopause means change of life and intuitively she did not want to admit. I told her bluntly that I would like to treat her on the lines of menopausal bleeding since in homeopathy, the treatment of excessive bleeding varies with age and personality unlike allopathy. I also stressed the point that clinical diagnosis at times is more important than the laboratory tests alone. She agreed and she was put on Trillium and Hammemelis and Millifolium – all mother tinctures and alternating with China 30. The bleeding came under control.

Reason

Most remedies were given on the principle of 'similar treats similar'.

I told her to throw away all the sophisticated and expensive allopathic preparations. She has gone back happily to USA and sent me a card of thanks.

OVARIAN CYSTS

Case I

A 21-year-old girl's parents phoned me that their daughter is having excruciating pain in lower abdomen. The surgeon and gynae-obs. nearby examined her and told that this is ovarian cyst and this should be operated upon immediately. They sought my advice and I also advised the same thing but they declined to have the operation done. Myself as a final year student of MBBS, remember that in the final exam, being given a case of ovarian cyst and asked about its complications, I told the examiner stangulation as one of the complications, so the patient should be operated upon. That impressed the examiner and she gave me good marks. So, in short, I explained to the parents of this girl but the very name of the operation frightened them. Next day ultrasound confirmed ovarian cyst and the gynae-obs. wanted to aspirate under ultrasound screening. Parents declined even that procedure.

Homeopathy

I gave combination A: (aco.+bell.+bry.+apis.) alternating with combination B: (cim.+colo.+cup.)

To my surprise, within a week, the whole thing melted like anything. She has been kept on a maintenance dose of Cimcifuga+Pulsatilla+Sepia for a few months, with infrequent dose of lachesis and thuja.

Reason

1. In acute condition with pain and inflammation, Aconite, Bell, and Bryonia is indispensable.
2. Apis is specific for ovary inflammation.
3. Cim, Colo and Cup.m acted like antispasmotic.
4. Hormonal control, the reason for which ovarian cyst developed, was controlled by Pulsatilla and Sepia.

STERILITY
(Infertility)

I have dealt with cases wherein **organic** cause in husband or wife has been excluded.

Case I

A Canadian, 28-year-old lady, married for the last 5 years, had no issue.

Allopathy

She went through all the modern investigations and

treatment, spending thousands of dollars, but did not conceive. Fertility drugs also did not help.

On my examination, I found that she was psychic, hysterical and trembling and had extreme degree of vaginismus, also having Dysparunea (painful intercourse).

I found that she had lot of thick cervical mucous secretions which were detrimental to the sperms. Also due to spasm of vagina, no semen was going into vagina.

Homeopathy & Reason

Staphy 30 alternate with Kali Phos 30, Avena Q once after meal for one week. Nat Carb 200 1 dose after 1 week. 3 months after my treatment, she became pregnant.
Staphy relieved spasm of vagina.
Nat Carb thinned the cervical mircus.

BREAST

In 21st century, this asset of women is assuming tremendous importance in the fashion world. It is essential to impress upon the fair sex and the men of different race and religion, certain myths and facts and misconceptions about this vital asset of a female body.

The following sentences may appear out of context of this book but in the light of cases (as mentioned below) it is imperative to mention apparently unpalatable (according to some) phrases.

Most men cannot put their finger on what is it they love about breasts. But majority will say it is their size, shape and texture. Just walk through any Egyptian artifacts, antiquities section of any museum, highly adorned breasts will be peeping out.

An average woman has 39.7 inches of breast, although there are variations in shape and size, which are normal in general. The following cases demonstrate my reasons for mentioning the details about this vital asset.

Case I

A 24-year-old West-European charming personality and a stunning beauty, who used to be a fashion model before, adopted a certain religion sect where it was prevailed upon them that breast is only for feeding the baby and not to be caressed or shown in provocative position even to their husbands. The girl became a hypochondriac, flattened her God-given gift with tight brassier, started hating the opposite sex.

I gave her the following few phrases which lifted her depression, anxiety and aversion to sex.

Female breast apart from breast feeding to the baby should be caressed by **men** in the following way:

1. TOUCH them like precious gems.
2. KISS them as if you have got a thirst that needs quenching.
3. LICK them lovingly like ice lollies.
4. TEASE them with gentle stokes.
5. SQUEEZE them like delicate juicy fruit.
6. SUCK them like sweeties.
7. BOUNCE them in your hands like little balls.

It took me two months of psychoanalysis and explaining the importance of breast and removing her religious insanity with homeopathy, she was a different girl, cheerful, social and full of love and affection.

Homeopathy

I gave her Sepia and Agnus.C in increasing potencies alongwith psychoanalysis and she became a normal woman in two months' time.

Case II

Many young and even married ladies do not know the normal variations of breasts. As a result of that, certain inferiority complexes creep in them and they run to Plastic surgeons or to Gynae-obstetricians.

Certain Important Facts

Human behaviour expert Desmond Morris explains the hidden meaning of breasts:

According to expert Susan Marchant-Haycox:

Men preferring small breasts are more independent and will do their own work.

Men preferring large breasts are confident and extrovert.

When aroused, female nipple length increases by upto 0.5 cm and the areola becomes deeper.

By orgasm, the breast of average female will have increased by 25% of its normal dimensions, becoming firmer and much more rounded.

British women have the biggest breast in Europe.

A young girl of 19 years came to me with severe anxiety that she may not be having cancer of the breast since the size of nipple on two sides is different. After explaining to her that it is a normal variation, she was relieved of her tension.

Case III

A young girl of 19 years was obsessed that her breast was very small (34) and her husband may leave her after her marriage because of her small breasts.

I reassured her and explained the normal variations and told her certain breast augmentation exercises. In addition, I gave her Sabal Serrulata-Q and Onosmodium in very high potencies. Her breasts' size increased to 36 in 4 months' time.

A.C.T.

Flat breasts, especially if associated with scanty periods, respond miraculously to Homeopathic treatment.

Allopathy

Commercialism in this particular field by plastic surgery has reached to such heights that both surgeons and patients had to repent for life. Surgeons have to repent if the things are not upto the expectation of the patient. Most of these patients suffer from inferiority complex. Patients have to suffer if things go wrong sooner or later. These days lot of cases are going in courts against the manufacturers. Recently, on my assignment in London, I was pained to learn how a 75-year-old plastic surgeon of a teaching hospital, retired 10 years ago, was sued by a patient because scars of incision for breast surgery (for cosmetic) were more prominent than the thin lines. The health authority had to pay damages of 1,32,000 pounds to the lady.

Homeopathy

Onosmodium in high potency given infrequently, followed by Sabal Serrulata 30 BD, changed the life of young girls with atrophic breasts.

If the girl has also weak eyesight and frontal headache along with atrophic breasts, Onosmodium is a boon but must be in high potency.

DYSPARUNEA
(Painful Coitus)

It is defined as painful intercourse. It is either in newly married couple owing to vaginismus making the vagina tight or at menopause owing to dryness of vagina caused by lower level of oestrogen hormones.

Allopathy

Allopathically, alprax in newly married couples, and lubricant jellies at menopause, both preparations intefere with orgasm and pleasure.

Homeopathy & Reason

Mag. phos, colocynth, staph. solve the problem like a miracle by acting as antispasmotic for vagina.

PAINFUL COITUS (Dysparunea)

After excluding any physical abnormalities both in men and women, if still there is painful coitus with no apparent cause, then the following treatment is often given.

Allopathy

Felt by men: Often the sexologists or the physicians give tranquilliser which interferes with performance of the act. Side-effect is worst than the disease.

Felt by women: If vaginismus is the cause, then Spasmotylic medicines like Spasmoproxyvon are given which dulls the mental sensation and interferes with the pleasure. If vaginitis is the cause, then various antifungal pessaries and local metroindozole preparations which cause irritation of tip of penis and sometimes severe allergic swelling of penis.

Homeopathy

For men: Sabal Serrulata-Q̇ and Selenium are very useful.

For women: If due to vaginismus, then Magnesium Phos 30 alternate with Gelsemium 30 and Ignatia 30. If due to vaginitis, then Sepia 30 alternating with Staphy 30 solves the problem.

PREGNANCY : ITS ACCOMPANYING AILMENTS

Abortion

1. Due to fright or fear.

Allopathy

Tranquillizers like Valium or Alzolam or Alprax are given by allopaths to prevent abortion.

Effect of Allopathy

The long-term side-effects of these tranquillizers on the foetus are unpredictable. The mother remains under constant fear, in case, these medications cause harmful effect on the baby. That fear itself is bad for the mother.

Homeopathy

Aconite 200, if given in time, often prevents abortion.

2. Due to false step or carrying heavy weight or other physical over-exertions.

Allopathy

Bruffen, Voveran, Diclofenal or Advil (U.S.A.).

Effect of Allopathy

These reduce the blood supply in the placenta, to the foetus and can have far-reaching consequences.

Homeopathy

In contrast to allopathy, Arnica 200 is an excellent remedy to prevent abortion.

3. Habitual abortion in 2nd, 3rd month.

Allopathy

Progesteron preparations are often given, which, at times, lead to other side-effects.

Homeopathy

Sabina is very good remedy, if there is pain in lower back and genitals, and blood is dark in colour.

Miscarriage

Specially in 8th month or when on delivery the baby dies soon after birth.

Allopathy

Tranquillizers, bed rest, Progesteron preparations.

Effect of Allopathy

I find this treatment often unsuccessful.

Homeopathy

In my experience:

(a) Viburnum Pru Q, if taken in time, has never let me down, provided the woman has faith in it.
(b) Sepia: If abortion occurs during 5th to 7th month with accompanying leucorrhoea and constipation, then Sepia is the best remedy.

Urinary Infection During Pregnancy

A.C.T.

Allopathy

Often antibiotics are given and caution is taken to prescribe the safest antibiotic which is not harmful to the foetus.

Effect of Allopathy

It is very common during pregnancy and at the same time antibiotic preparations like Norflox or Lommef have tremendous side-effects, when given during pregnancy.

Homeopathy

Cantharis 30, alternating with Berberis Q, gives excellent results. If still there is no improvement in symptoms, then Apis M 200 is also added to the above homeopathic treatment.

Vomiting (Morning Sickness)

Allopathy

Domstal and Perinorm are the standard preparations.

Effect of Allopathy

The effects of these are on extrapyramidal symptoms. Perinorm should not be given if there is history of epilepsy.

Homeopathy

Nux Vomica alternate with Ant Crud 6. Colchicum, if smell of food brings nausea in addition to vomiting. In incessant and resistant type of nausea, Symphoricarpus racel in 200 dilution is the head remedy.

Aversion

There is no treatment in allopathy for this symptom of pregnancy.

Homeopathy

For aversion to bread, Sepia is the main remedy.

Bearing Down (Prolapse)

Allopathy

Pessaries are given during pregnancy, or the foot side of the bed is raised.

Effect of Allopathy

Pessaries can lead to infection. Positioning of the bed with foot side raised can lead to reflux oesophagitis and breathlessness.

Homeopathy

Sepia 30, 200 is an excellent remedy apart from the fact that it helps in pregnancy just like Progesteron preparation in pregnancy.

Breathing (Breathlessness)

Difficult breathing during pregnancy.

Allopathy

Often Deriphylline and other Bronchodilator preparations are given.

Effect of Allopathy

These cause insomnia, tremors and gastritis.

Homeopathy

It is a tailor-made treatment. Nux Vomica is very helpful.

Cough

Hundreds of pregnant women have been referred to me by gynae-obs. for this symptom since allopathic medicines are not advisable to be given owing to side-effects on foetus.

Homeopathy

1. Kali Brom in reflex cough, dry fatiguing cough at night.
2. Causticum : Dry cough.
3. Conium : Cough on mental or physical exertion.

Fear of Death During Pregnancy

Allopathy

Alprax or Alzolam or Vallium are often the medicines prescribed.

Effect of Allopathy

Long-term side-effects on foetus. Moreover, it is contra-indicated in pregnancy. Hypotension sometimes occurs, which is dangerous for the foetus.

Homeopathy

Aconite 200, 4 hourly is best suited for fear of pregnancy.

Taste

Changes during pregnancy. There is hardly anything in allopathy to offer.

Homeopathy

a. Desire for salt or salted food: Natrum mur.
b Desire for unusual articles of food: Helidonium.
c. Desire for earth or chalk: Nitric Acid.
d. Desire for sugar or pickles: Sulphur.

Oedema

During pregnancy, especially of feet or whole body, it is very common.

Allopathy

Often diuretics like Lasix or Dytide are given.

Effect of Allopathy

Weakness follows by taking these diuretics because of loss of minerals, calcium and potassium. Replacement of potassium causes acidity on a pre-existing acidity due to pressure of uterus on the stomach.

Homeopathy

1. Apis m 200, 6 hourly is an excellent remedy.
2. Ars. alb., if there is associated heart trouble.

Foetus Displacement

Allopathy

In some cases, Gynae. and Obst. are able to correct the position in early stage, but I have seen that while doing this procedure, patient goes into abortion or bleeding P.V. or interference in the blood supply to the placenta.

Homeopathy

Pulsatilla is an excellent remedy for putting the foetus or the child in right place.

Foetus Movement

a. If movements have ceased.	Caulophyllum.30
b. If movements are violent and painful and disturb the sleep of mother with urge to urinate.	Thuja 30
c. Sensitiveness, tenderness and soreness is felt in uterus on account of movements of foetus.	Arnica 200

Insanity During Pregnancy

Allopathy

Most of the allopathic drugs are tranquillisers and anti-depressants. These are associated with disastrous side-effects both to the mother and child. Never forget the disaster done by Thalidamide in the western world in the 70's.

Homeopathy

Stramonium 200.

Cramp and Pain in Abdomen and Legs During Pregnancy

Allopathy

Anti-inflammatory and pain killers are not advisable since these only relieve the symptoms without treating the cause.

Homeopathy

Viburnum Op. Q is excellent for cramps and pain in abdomen and legs.

Sleeplessness

Tranquillisers are not advisable owing to their side-effects.

Homeopathy

Anacardium 200 – morning.
Coffea – 200 at bed time.
If it is due to fear or grief or sadness, then Aconite 200.

Toothache

During pregnancy, it is very common.

Allopathy

Advil (USA), Bruffen, Flexon, or Combiflam, Voveran are not advisable since these cause:

1. Fluid retention on an already oedematous lady.
2. Skin or asthmatic reactions are very common.

Homeopathy

Staphy 30, 200 alternating with Spigelia 30. If no relief with Staphysagria or Spigelia, then Sepia is main remedy for toothache during pregnancy.

Urine (Retention)

Frequent desire to urinate. Urine escapes in a few drops before reaching the vessel.

Allopathy

Often the catheter is placed in the bladder. This very often leads to urinary infection.

Homeopathy

Causticum alternating with Sepia never fails to cure it.

ATROPHY OF NIPPLES AND BREAST

A.C.T.

Obviously this creates psychological problem in the women or girls at puberty.

Allopathy

Plastic surgery is not successful in all cases, apart from the cost of such operations. At times, the results of such operations are worse than the original disease. Many such cases have been reported recently in the press in U.K. where patients are complaining about leaking transplants a few years after implantation.

Homeopathy

1. If the sexual desire is also less with slow development of breast at puberty, then Conium is often successful.
2. If the girl has excessive sleep tendency with incarcerated flatus, then Nux mos. 30 works the trick.

BIRTH CONTROL

A.C.T.

It is needless to discuss the merits and demerits of different allopathic means of birth control in this book.

Allopathy

Everybody is familiar with the potential dangers of contraceptive pills. Each woman reacts differently to these pills. Blood pressure, deep venous thrombosis of legs and vision could be affected due to these pills. However, it is of interest to mention that recently quinine preparations were locally used as contraceptive which act as irritants and cause scarring, thus leading to prevention of conception by mechanical means. But many cases of cancer of cervix have been reported with this method of contraception.

Homeopathy

Without any side-effects I have prescribed the following treatment with success:

1. In 90% of the cases, Natrum Mur 200 taken on 1st, 2nd and 3rd day after cessation of monthly course. These dosages must be repeated after every mense till conception is not desired.
2. Pulsatilla 200, one dose daily for 4 days, continuously before the regular date of menstruation, will be sufficient to prevent conception.

5

Urinary Diseases

ACUTE CYSTITIS

It is one of the very common annoying ailments affecting especially women owing to anatomical difference in the urethra from that in men.

Common symptoms are burning, stranguary and frequency of micturition.

Allopathy

Antibiotics, especially Norflox and other related antibiotics of this group, often help dramatically.

Effect of Allopathy

Vaginal fungal infection as a result of the use of broadspectrum antibiotics is very common. This causes itching which leads to urinary infection. So a vicious circle sets up. **Cystitis causes vaginitis and vaginitis causes cystitis.**

Homeopathy

Cantharis 30 and Berberis Q alternating with each other help a lot. But the main part played by homeopathy is:
a. In recurrent and relapse of chronic cystitis.

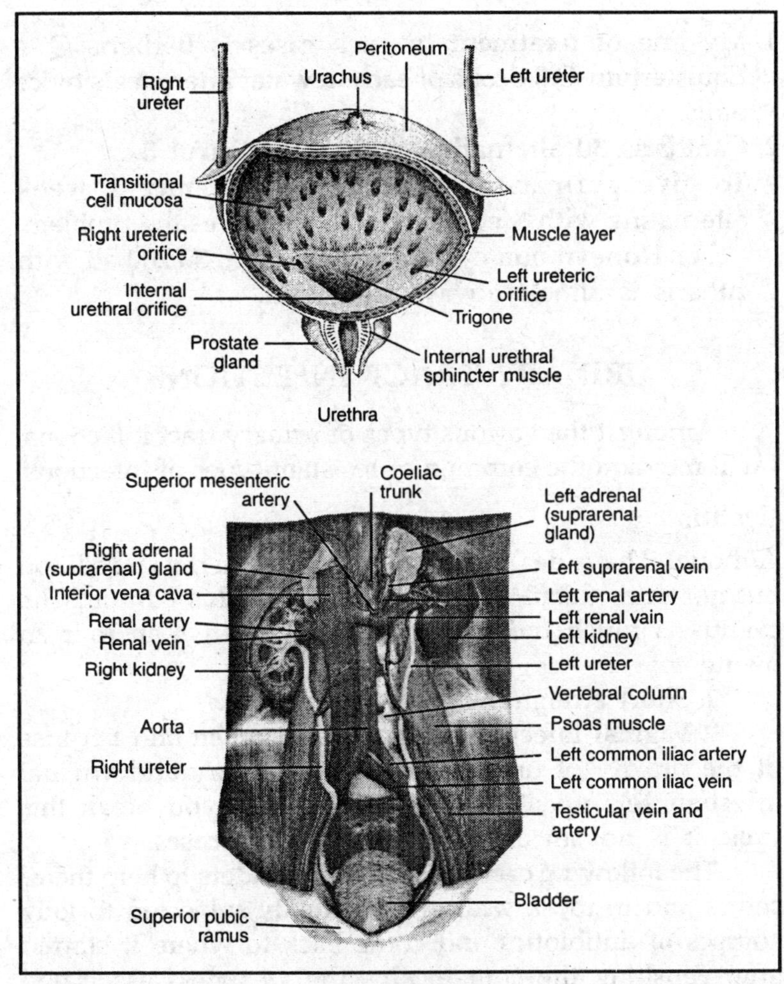

Urinary System

b. Where culture report is negative but the patient still suffers from symptoms of cystitis.

c. Patient has become resistant to most of the antibiotics or gets allergic reaction. In **chronic** recurrent cases, allopathy has hardly anything to offer except in cases of surgical cause or congenital cause.

1. My line of treatment in such cases is Berberis Q + Equisterium-Q 5 drops of each in water after meals twice daily.
2. Cantharis 30 alternating with Sabal Serrul 3x.

To give permanent cure, Thuja 200 once a week alternating with Medorrhanium 200 solves the problem.

For **Honeymoon** cystitis, I find Staph, 30,200 alt with Cantharis is almost always successful.

URINARY TRACT INFECTIONS

Amongst the various types of urinary tract infections, I will mention the common or resistant types of infections.

Cystitis

Although I have dealt with on this subject in my last edition but not in as detail as I will mention in this edition. The cystitis is much more common in women than in men owing to:

1 Short straight urethra.

2 Vaginal infection, common in women and because of the proxity of urethra to vagina, urinary and vaginal infection sets up a vicious cycle. Unless you break this cycle it is not an easy job to cure such cases.

The following cases will help the readers to help themselves and to those who are repeatedly subjected to long courses of antibiotics and come back to where it started after finishing the course, plus the weakness associated with antibiotics.

NOCTURNAL POLYURIA IN WOMEN

The urine tests in such cases are often normal. There is no uterine tumour to cause pressure on urinary bladder.

Allopathy

Antibiotics are hardly of any use to cure these cases permanently.

Homeopathy

Murex 30 alternating with Sabal Serrul 3x for 2 weeks. Alfa Q + Avena Q BD after meals.

INCONTINENCE OF URINE
(Uncontrollable Urination)

It is very common in women than men after the age of 40 to 50.

In women, since the urethra is small in length and straight, apart from other factors like delayed labour and multiple pregnancies which affect the sphincter.

In men, the common cause is enlarged prostate or prostatitis.

In both the sexes, symptoms of frequency, urgency and occasionally burning and pain (if infection supervenes) are there.

If investigations like ultrasound, repeated urine culture and PSA (Antigenic test for prostate) are all normal, and patients still continue to have symptoms, then Homeopathy has a strong role to play.

Allopathy

In the following cases, I am dealing with those where repeated courses of norflox and 4th generation of floxacine have failed to control the symptoms permanently.

Homeopathy

1. Cantharis and Causticum (in different potencies) often succeed in controlling the symptoms.

However, I have seen a very resistant case where I had to give Terebinth after giving one dose of Thuja 200, before the symptoms came under control. In this case, all urine reports were normal. Equestrium Q is of unquestionable value.

In stubborn cases of prostate, infrequent doses of Thuja and Baryta carb are of immense value.

I must emphasise the point that sometimes with no diabetes or urine infection, frequency of micturition is due to hyperacidity of stomach. I could control this with nux vomica and natrum phos.

Cases I, II, III

I have seen many cases of prostate being unnecessarily operated upon if they had slight symptoms of urinary problem, after catheterisation (done for some or the other reason). The infection invariably supervenes following catheterisation. Even after the catheter is out, there is some degree of prostatitis and the greed of surgeon leads to the decision of surgery, especially if the ultrasound shows slight degree of hypertrophy, which would be there in any case. I appreciate the need for surgery in really enlarged prostate causing severe symptoms or suspected malignancy.

It is very common in **women** at menopause. After excluding organic causes like uterine tumour, prolapse Uterus, urinary infection it comes as a challenge to urologist to cure such cases.

I have seen hundreds of women with this malady after spending hundreds of dollars on investigations, still having problem, when every investigation is normal.

Homeopathy

Causticum 30, 200, 1M has never let me down. It has not only cured control of urine but also any associated complaints of arthritis and spondylitis.

Ambra 30, 200 is another excellent remedy which by curing itching of vagina, indirectly cures aseptic cystitis and thus takes control of micturition. In my experience caladium does not help.

In **men**, the common cause is Prostatitis with enlarged prostate. I have described its treatment already in the preceding chapters.

PROSTATE

Benign prostatic hypertrophy (prostate enlargement) is also a common problem. Prostatic enlargement commonly occurs after the age of 45.

Symptoms of prostatic enlargement include frequent need for urination, especially at night, interrupted urination or incomplete emptying of bladder, burning or painful urination and frequent bladder infections. Many patients may notice trouble in urination, a weak stream or dribbling after urination. If you have enlarged prostate, PSA (prostate specific antigen) level may be high.

Allopathy

Surgery is often recommended and can be effective. But surgery can result in incontinence and ejaculatory dysfuntion and, at times, impotency.

Homeopathy

The correct homeopathy can reverse the symptoms of prostate enlargement, without the need for surgical intervention.

Prostate Cancer

It is very common in the west than in the east. The early symptoms of prostate cancer are similar to prostate enlargement. The PSA may be or may not be high. Some prostate cancers are symptomless, while others can be life threatening.

A.C.T.

Homeopathy

It is important to mention that apart from some general remedies for enlarged prostate, some remedies are specific with each case.

As per my experience, I will mention **Conium** as the head remedy. The characteristic symptom of conium is too frequent or dribbling. It is interrupted, stops when straining, then flows when relaxed.

Baryta carb is another remedy which solves so many problems in an elderly person when given for enlarged prostate. It controls the high blood pressure, in addition to preventing degeneration of the body tissues.

Ferrum picricum is an excellent remedy as illustrated in the following case. Apart from controlling senile prostate hypertrophy, it improves the nerve deafness and warts, if any, present in old age.

Sabal Serrulata-Q is unquestionable in senile enlarged prostate.

Case I

A 60-year-old man came to me with symptoms of frequent urination, had to wait for some time before he could pass dribbling urination. He has been taking Sabal Serrulata-Q on his own but significant relief.

Examination and ultrasound revealed prostate hypertrophy. He also complained of sensory-neural deafness and his neck was full of warts. He had also impotency.

I started treatment with Thuja 200, to be given once a week and on remaining days, I gave combination of ferrum picicum, baryta carb and conium.

To my surprise, he started showing tremendous improvement not only in urination but also in hearing as well as of warts. My this combination of remedies acted as multiprong attack on all his ailments.

Case II

A man, 65 years old, came with history of flatulence and occasional bleeding per rectum. He also had urinary symptoms of enlarged prostate (dribbling, frequent and occasionally burning). The symptoms used to get aggravated whenever he took spicy food.

I treated him on two counts:

a. Bleeding piles with hammemalis and aesculus.
b. Prostate enlargement and prostatis with causticum, baryta carb and ferrum picric.

He felt 80% improvement in two weeks in most of his symptoms.

Conclusion

It is very essential to treat cases of piles, if these are there, with associated enlarged prostate. In my experience, these are often there.

PROSTATITIS AND HYPERTROPHY OF THE PROSTATE

Although there are a lot of advances in surgical field for the cure of this ailment by T.U.R. and Laser, as a result of which there are less bleeding, less chances of infection, and short stay in the hospital, but certain complications like 1. Catheteric infection, and 2. Enuresis (no control of urine), or 3. Anaesthetic complications in old age should not be underestimated.

Homeopathy

My homeopathic treatment in such cases:

1. Populis Tremuloides 30 alternating with Sabal Serrulata 3x.
2. Equisterium Q, 5-8 drops in water after meals.

The following case illustrates the perils of allopathic treatment and life saving measures of homeopathy:

Case

A topmost physician was operated upon by an Urologist of repute in the capital. Hell broke to the poor physician when he got catheteric infection which resulted in incontinence. Latest antibiotics imported as an emergency measure brought the infection under control, but reduced the platelet level to a dangerous level resulting in Haematuria, extreme prostration, anaemia and severe depression. There was no scope left to give any more allopathy. At this stage, when he was bedridden, I was consulted and my following line of treatment helped him:

1. Kali Phos 30 + Anacardium 30 replaced his heavy doses of allopathic tranquillizers. It controlled depression as well.
2. Populus Treumloids 30 and Sabal Serrulata 3x and Equistereum 3x controlled all urinary symptoms.
3. Later, after urinary symptoms were brought under control, I gave China 30 + Nux Vomica 30 + Carbo Veg 30 for his debility.

FREQUENT URINATION IN MEN

The following paragraphs exclude the causes of excessive urination due to venereal or non-venereal causes due to infections which should be treated on the lines of proper antibiotics depending upon the culture and sensitivity.

In elderly people, (aged 50 onwards) the common cause is either enlarged prostate or prostatitis. But chronic prostatitis often leads to hypertrophy of the prostate.

After excluding any associated urinary infection by culture and sensitivity and treating accordingly, if the symptoms of enlarged prostate and frequent micturition still persist, then homeopathy plays excellent role in the majority of cases.

Case I

A 65-year-old man, with clinical symptoms of hypertrophy of prostate with frequent micturition, has been put on hythaltone for his high blood pressure and for enlarged prostate. However, he started getting the side-effects of the drug leading to too much lowering of blood pressure. As a result, I gave him the following homeopathic drugs:

Homeopathy

1. Sabal serrulata-Q + Equestrium-Q: 8 drops three times a day after meals.

2. Once in two weeks he was given Baryta carb 200 alternating with Thuja 200 (once in two weeks).
3. Combination of Ferrum-picic+Causticum and Apis was given in the form of pills three times a day everyday.
4. It took me three months to make him symptom-free.

FREQUENT URINATION IN WOMEN

This is a common complaint occuring in women under the following conditions:

1. After caesarean without any injury to the bladder.
2. At menopause.
3. In Vulvovaginitis.

In dealing with above causes, I am excluding diabetes, diuretics and some antihypertensive drugs which cause excessive urination.

In excessive urination in men, I will deal under different heading.

After Caesarean

It may be after a few weeks or even months that the patient starts getting this symptom. It is due to weakness of the urinary bladder symptom owing to manipulation of the viscera at the time of operation. It can also happen in prolonged labour.

Homeopathy

In such cases, I find Causticum is of unquestionable value giving miraculous results.

At Menopause

It occurs at this phase of life partly due to shrinking of muscles leading to weakness of the sphincter and also due to hypersensitivity of control of the bladder owing to itching in the surrounding vagina due to dryness.

Homeopathy

Alumina, Calcarea fluor, and Ambra have never let me down.

Vulvovaginitis: It is advisable to treat this condition with antifungal preparations with allopathy, but these creams should not contain steroids or hormones. I find simple imidil, vaginal pessaries work very well. However, in advance cases, Flucanazole preparations may have to be given by mouth.

BED WETTING

It is one of the most annoying ailments, especially to the parents of the child and also to the child itself.

Allopathy

Various suggestions like waking up the child during night, not drinking water before going to bed, electronic alarms are of hardly any use.

Homeopathy

Equisterium Q, 5-8 drops, 2-3 times a day in half a cup of water.

E. COLI : URINARY INFECTION

A.C.T.

It is one of the commonest ailments, especially amongst women, more so near menopause. It is a challenge to the Urologists all over the world.

Allopathy

Commonly, physicians give antibiotics according to culture and sensitivity, patient gets relief and culture comes negative after the course of antibiotics.

Effect of Allopathy

A couple of weeks after stopping the antibiotics, the infection comes back. Commonly, Floxacine group of antibiotics from 1st to 4th generation are given. Repeated Gastrointestinal disturbances, pseudomembranous colitis, headache, blurred vision, joint pains, Tachycarida, Stevens-Johnson syndrome are caused due to antibiotics.

Case

A young Kashmiri girl came to me with severe U.T.I. with 60 pus cells and blood count TLC 2500. After repeated use of antibiotics, she was extremely debilitated.

Homeopathy

Berberis Q, Equisetum and Cantharis 30 controlled the symptoms in 24 hours. This treatment was carried on for 3 weeks and the patient got completely cured for her debility and extreme prostration. I gave her Carbo Veg 200, 1M Selenium 200 and Acid Phos. 30, 200. Vitamins could not be given since she was allergic to vitamins.

STERILITY IN MALES

If there is Azoospermia or Oligospermia associated with or without impotency, in allopathy, often testicular biopsy is done and it is more often normal. Even if it shows oligospermia with sluggish sperms, the treatment often given is Testosteron hormones under one or other brand names. The accompanying side-effects and danger of cancer of prostate are there with testosteron.

Homeopathy

Damiana Q, Sabal Serrulata Q and Conium 200, 1M often succeeds in curing sterility and impotency.

B. COLI INFECTION

B. Coli Infection of urinary passages is a bugbear to surgeons, gynae-obstetricians and urologists. I am sure they cannot deny that recurrence is notorious even after giving repeated doses of broad spectrum antibiotics.

Allopathy

Norflox, Lomeflox will do a wonderful job in acute infections, but one of the common side-effects is vaginal and ear fungal infections.

Homeopathy

I have successfully treated antibiotic resistant cases with the following:

1. Thuja 1M once a week and then once a month.
2. Berberis Q 10 drops in a cup of warm water every 3 hours.
3. B. Coli in 30 potency is very useful.

STRICTURE OF URETHRA

This is quite a common condition in both sexes. In women, it often occurs after repeated deliveries with prolonged labour or too frequent and prolonged catheterisation.

In men the common cause is either past history of venereal disease or prostate involvement. The common symptom is tendency of frequent but small quantity of urine.

Allopathy

Often dilatation by passing bougies is the line of treatment. In men prostate operation (if that is the cause) by laser is preferable.

If allopathy fails as often in case of dilatation by bougies, then Homeopathy plays a significant role:

Homeopathy

1. Staphysagaria 30,200 is successful in majority of cases.
2. Clematis.E 30,200 is very often helpful especially in resistant and post-gonococcal cases.
3. In other cases, Causticum and Thiosinamun 30,200 are successful.

URAEMIA

Very high level of urea due to kidney failure for one or other reason is the common cause.

Allopathy

In such cases, often dialysis is the first line of treatment. But in India, poor facilities and high cost along with the threat of AIDS and Hepatitis B, pose a great problem.

Homeopathy

I have treated such cases in advance renal failure secondary to malignant hypertension, C.H.F. and liver failure.

1. Apis 30,200.
2. Urea 6,30.
3. Stropanthus-Q, which acts as diuretic also.
4. Cuprum -Arsenicum 3x in resistant cases.

6

Digestive System (Gastroenterology)

COLITIS

It is inflammation of colon, also called Chronic Dysentery. It is often caused by bacterial infection (Entamoeba histolytica) which destroys the intestinal wall leading to Ulcerative Colitis or Amoebic Colitis. Patient often has lower abdominal pain with passage of blood mucous and urging of stools soon after eating, because pressure of food or gas formed in the congested colon cause frequent urging of stools. Second common cause is Giardiasis caused by micro-organism called Giardia. This condition is common in children throughout the world, especially in Asian countries. Common symptoms are nausea, loss of appetite, abdominal pain, slimy stools mixed with indigested food.

ULCERATIVE COLITIS

This condition is becoming very common all over the world. Nobody knows the exact cause, the common theories are amoebic colitis or stress and strain of modern life. Irritable bowel syndrome (I.B.S.) is considered to be the precursor of ulcerative colitis.

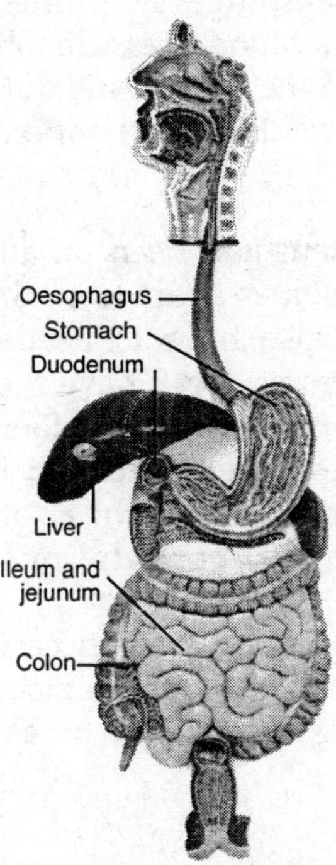

Digestive System

Allopathy

On the basis of these theories, the treatment is done accordingly.

In Asian countries, the common cause is Amoebiasis, hence Metrogyl and Tinidazole preparations are the common line of treatment.

In western countries, mental stress and strain are the common cause of this disease. Hence, tranquillizers are given.

However, since there is inflammation of bowel, anti-inflammatory drugs like tegretal and steroids, both locally and systemically are the common line of treatment.

A.C.T.

I have seen such innumerable patients who had only symptomatic relief with such drugs and have landed with side-effects of steroids (cushing's syndrome: bull's neck, facial hair in women, high blood pressure, obesity, diabetes and kidney changes) and the disease still not cured, only treated symptomatically and that too temporarily.

Homeopathy

The longer the patient had been on allopathic drugs, the more difficult it becomes apart from the fact that complications of steroids also have to be dealt with.

Another depressing fact I have seen is that allopaths keep pushing iron preparations, whether these are absorbed or not, whether these are assimilated in the body or not and I have seen cases of iron cirrhosis of liver due to heavy doses for prolonged periods pushing these iron preparations.

My line of treatment in such cases is as below, the potency and the changes in the remedies is governed by the condition and age of the patient, also other conditions associated with it.

1. Bleeding:

Often I give in **two combinations** alternating with each other.

(a) Hammelis+Millefolium+Trillium.

Reason

Hammemelis is antihaemmorhagic in pelvic region bleeding. Millefolium has a general anti-haemmorhagic effect. Trillium is specific of menopausal bleeding.

(b) China+Acid phos+Carboveg

Reason

Apart from antihaemmorhagic effect of China, this is the head remedy in loss of vital fluids alongwith acid phos which has a magic effect in regaining energy in the event of loss of fluids. Carboveg apart from recouping the patient controls the residual venous congestion.

2. Ulceration, flatulence, loose motions:

(a) Merc sol+Aloe+Nitric acid; (b) Colchicum+Colocynth+ Mag. phos.

The above combinations have never let me down. Often these patients are anaemic, so Ferrum phos 6x or Ferrium 5 often helps to build up haemoglobin.

Case I

A young lady doctor, daughter of renowned doctor parents, was suffering for the last five years from ulcerative colitis. She was being treated by topmost gastroenterologists of Delhi with heavy doses of steroids, both internally and by colonoscopy, still bleeding, and developed cushing's syndrome.

Important thing to note is that with all this ulcerative colitis, allopaths were giving her oral iron preparations and at times anti-inflammatory drugs for pain which used to aggravate her condition. I had to give her iron injection to quicken the haemoglobin formation.

The other important point to note is that repeated courses of metrogyl preparation cause aseptic inflammation of intestine.

It is very essential that diet in such cases should be bland and devoid of spices and should be supplemented with isabgol husk.

MUCOUS-ULCERATIVE COLITIS

A.C.T.

Recurring pain in abdomen with constipation or diarrhoea and lot of mucous. It is more common in the West than in the East due to more stress and strain in the west. I must emphasise that in any type of colitis, it is not necessary that stools will show a positive E. Histolytica or Giardia Cyst.

Allopathy

Flagyl, Metrogyl, Tiniba, Valium, Alzolam, Larpose and Steroids (systemic and locally).

A.C.T.

Effect of Allopathy

These allopathic medicines have very adverse effects. The depressing fact is that these drugs do not cure. When they are discontinued, symptoms recur in a short time again. Adverse effects are: metallic taste, mouth ulcer, loss of appetite, inflammation of intestinal wall, gastritis, blood changes. Steroids cause dreadful side-effects after continued use (hirsuitisis, obesity, high blood pressure, high blood sugar, menstrual disturbances).

The following cases will demonstrate the miraculous and curing result of Homeopathic treatment for Ulcerative Colitis.

Case I

A doctor's wife from U.K. came with ulcerative colitis due to prolonged use of Tegretol for migrain. She was on steroids enema, systemic intake of steroids for colitis from time to time. Haemostatic medicines like Dicynene were used for rectal bleeding.

Homeopathy

I gave mixture of A, B and C in cyclic rotation as below:

A. BlumiaQ + Ficus ReligiosaQ+Hamme.Q

B. Puls.30+Merc cor30

C. China30+Colocynth 30+Mag.phos 30+Cup.met 30

To give her permanent cure I gave a few doses of Thuja 200 at 1 weeks' interval.

Case II

A 34-year-old German lady, wife of a Diplomat, came to me. She had tried everything for Amoebic Colitis from topmost Gastro-enterologists but got no permanent cure. I gave "Kutazaristha" for 2 weeks and she had no more recurrences, as she stayed 2 years more in India after my treatment.

Her child was also suffering from Amoebiasis but he did not take "Kutazaristha" since the taste of Ayurvedic preparation is horrible.

Homeopathy

I gave the child Emetine 30 alternate with Ipecac 200 for 1 week. Then I gave Emetine 200 once a week and Sulphur 200 once a week in cyclic order.

Case III

A British Anaesthetist colleague of mine often used to be off work owing to ulcerative colitis.

Allopathy

She told me she had tried everything (Steroids, Tranquillisers, Flagyl), but it recurred. On my suggestion to try Homeopathy for her ulcerative colitis, she laughed. Anyhow, after a month when she was suffering badly, she said that she could have a trial of Homeopathy.

A.C.T.

Homeopathy

I gave her Avena Q + Alstonia (1:1), Merc Cor 200 alternating with Ipec 200. She was free from the symptoms for a month but it recurred again. Then I gave Sulphur 200. She was better for a while but it relapsed after six weeks. I asked her if she loves her cat very much. She said, "Of course, we eat together in the same dish." I asked bluntly to get her cat examined by a Vet. It was found that the cat had severe degree of Amoebiasis.

A.C.T.

Case IV

This case demonstrates the importance of **examination** in Homeopathy also. A lady, 45 years old, interior designer by profession, requested me if I could give her medicine for her colitis on the telephone and that she will send the fees by post as she is too busy to come to the clinic. I told her that Allopathy has no cure for ulcerative colitis. She knew this fact, since she had already tried three topmost Gastroenterologists of the world during her visits abroad, but got no improvement. She also said, "Do you have to examine me even for giving Homeopathy." She had been taking medicines for six months from a Homeopath who never examined her but used to give treatment simply on asking questions. I will only say, "God save the patients from such Homeopaths who never examine the patients." It reminds me of more cases, though not in the same context of colitis, of not examining the patient. A 40-year-old lady was being treated for deafness and noises in the ear for six months. I asked, "Has the doctor examined her ears?" She said, "Yes, he examined the ears with a torch and said that there is congestion." I fail to understand how such Homeopaths can see the ears without auroscope. Then there is no difference in quacks sitting at railway platforms and such Homeopaths. I removed hard wax from this patient's ear and in one sitting, patient got cured.

During the lifetime of Father of Homeopathy, there were not much diagnostic facilities available. Due to advancement in diagnostic facilities, these should be utilised to the best advantage of the patient in arriving at correct diagnosis in the light of clinical symptoms.

DIARRHOEA AND VOMITING

It is especially common in India owing to hot weather with poor hygienic conditions, making ideal culture for Diarrhoea and Dysentery.

Allopathy

For Diarrhoea and Dysentery, often Gram-Neg, Gramogyl, Dependal M and Immosec, Ciplox, Metrogyl, Ciplox ct are the drugs given.

A.C.T.

Effect of Allopathy

Gramogyl and Metrogyl are notorious for causing mouth

ulcers, loss of appetite and severe headache. Ciplox usually given for Bacillary type of Dysentery should not be given to persons below the age of 16 years as it hampers the growth. Loss of appetite is another side-effect and if the patient is having Diarrhoea and Dysentery along with loss of appetite due to the medication, it leads to dehydration.

Metronidazole given for Amoebiasis + Giardiasis under one or other different patent names (Tiniba, Fasygin) are most harmful for causing Gastritis and Stomatitis (mouth ulcers). Then Ranitidine preparations are given to counteract acidity. Ranitidine causes constipation.

I emphatically say that long term use of Metroindazole preparations cause weakness of intestine and poor absorption of food. Most of the pain-killers given for one or other conditions cause Diarrhoea.

Antibiotics very often cause Diarrhoea and Vomiting by disturbing the useful bacteria (lactobacil).

Homeopathy

In contrast, homeopathy:

1. Cures the patient permanently.
2. Increases the digestive power of stomach and resistance of intestines.
3. Remedy acts very specifically depending upon the cause, as given below:

Acute Diarrhoea due to:

1. Polluted water and ice-cream	Ars.alb. 6, 30 Alstonia Q
2. Teething	Chamomilla 6, 30 Ars.alb. 6
3. Fatty food	Puls.30
4. Allopathic drugs	Carb.veg 30, Nux. vom. 30, Nit. acid
5. Vomiting and Diarrhoea	Ipecac 30, 200 and Veratrum alb 200 1M
6. Debility and weakness	Carbo Veg 30 + China 30
7. Summer Diarrhoea	Croton tr. 30

Chronic Diarrhoea due to:
Colitis,
Giardiasis and
Amoebiasis.

Allopathy

Often the medicines given are: Metronidazole, Secnil Tiniba, Fasygin, Gramogyl. These are notorious for increased acidity, skin reaction, headache. I feel these preparations cause non-infective colitis and make the patient permanent case of ulcerative colitis. Interestingly, we allopaths give these preparations for colitis.

Homeopathy

Ipecac 200 alternate with Emetine 200, both twice a day. To give permanent cure, Sulphur 200 and Natrum Sulph 200 each once in a fortnight.

CONSTIPATION

Insufficient food, less fluid intake or food with low roughage or certain medicines, like Isoptin, cause constipation.

Allopathy

Dulcolax, Milk of Magnesia, Cremaffin and Lactulose are the common drugs given for constipation.

Effect of Allopathy

Constipation is worst after taking these laxatives and purgatives. These are also habit-forming.

Homeopathy

Homeopathy is very specific as given below:

1. Constipation in children. : Alumina 30, Nux Vom 200, Bryonia 30.

2. Constipation due to abuse of purgatives.	:	Hydrastasis 30, Nux Vom 200.
3. Constipation in heavy dieting people.	:	Nux Vom, sulphur.
4. Constipation with sedentary habits. (long hours of sitting)	:	Aletris, Collin, Nux. vom.
5. Constipation during pregnancy.	:	Sepia 30, Podo.30
6. Constipation in old age.	:	Plat, Alum, Opium, Avena.
7. Constipation in travellers.	:	Alum.Hydrastasis. Nux. vom.
8. Constipation due to weakness of intestines and rectum, weakness due to the use of Allopathic drugs like antacids, pain-killers.	:	Aes 30, Aloe 30, Alf Q + Ave Q + Aletris Q – 10-15 drops BD after meals.
9. Constipation due to nervous, excitable, weak, acidic temperament.	:	Ambra 30 alt. with Arg Nit 30 2-3 times a day.
10. Chronic constipation of years standing (easily tired, weak, sinking, sensation as if stools are forcing down the lower part of bowel, weak peristalsis).	:	Hydrastasis 30, Aletris Q, morning and evening after meals.

Case

Out of thousands, I give the history of one very senior G.P. suffering from constipation for the last many years. He has tried everything, e.g., Trifla Churan and other Herbolax, but no relief. I cured his obstinate constipation with the prescription of :

Homeopathy

Lycopodium 200 alternate days, Hydrastasis Q, 5 drops, BD after meals.

In other very resistant cases, I had to give Sulphur 200, one dose a week to give permanent cure.

GASTRITIS

Acute Gastritis

Usually follows irritating food: allopathic drugs like NSAID, Alcohol, stress.

Allopathy

Ranitidine or its derivatives like ocid, omnaprazole.

A.C.T.

Effect of Allopathy

Dryness of mouth and constipation.

Homeopathy

ARG. Nit 30 alternate with Ars alb 30 and Bismuth 6,30.

Chronic Gastritis

It is common amongst people taking spicy food and lot of chillies, pickles, smoking, alcohol. Sometimes chronic gastritis present with loss of appetite and flatulence.

Allopathy

Cispride, Zanetac, Omnaprazol (Ocid).

A.C.T.

Effect of Allopathy

Increase in Haemorrhoids (Piles) is the common side-effect with Cispride, Zanetac causes dryness and constipation. Omnaprazole can lead to Achlorohydria. Cysapride could be dangerous to heart (arrythmias).

Homeopathy

Nux Vom 30 (if diarrhoea)
Nux Vom 200 (if constipation)
Carbo Veg 30 alternate with China 30.
Hydrastasis 30 BD
Chionanthus Q, 5 drops after meals

REFLUX OESOPHAGITIS

This condition is becoming increasingly common and since its symptoms mimic of angina, cervical spondylosis, and heart attack, all investigations are essential to rule out other sinister conditions before labelling diagnosis of reflux oesophagitis.

After the diagnosis of reflux oesophagitis is confirmed, often the following treatment is advised by gastroenterologists.

Allopathy

1. **Antacids** like ranitidine, pantoprazole, ocid, omez acting on proton pump.
2. **Properistaltic drugs** like domstal and perinorm.
3. **Neutralising antacids** like digene, gellusil and mucain gel.
4. **General preventive measures:**

a. Not to lie soon after meals.
b. Do not overload stomach.
c. Avoid chillies and spicy food.
d. Reduce weight.

A.C.T.

Following are the adverse and side-effects of the above drugs which brought many patients to me for homeopathic treatment:

1. All groups of antacids cause extreme dryness of throat, leading to hoarseness and if the medical practitio-

ner is unaware of this side-effect, he might give decongestant and antihistaminic for hoarseness, as I have seen very often.

Recently, the case came to me as an emergency who was almost getting choked with thick tenacious and viscous saliva almost lying at laryngeal opening leading to suffocation. I immediately sucked the salivary secretions, and stopped all antacids and gave him homeopathic and steam inhalation and plenty of fluids and homeopathy for acidity which was due to antibiotics which the doctor has given to him.

He heaved a sigh of relief within 24 hours.

The other common side-effects with antacids is whether proton type or neutralizing type, these cause constipation and gastric upset. Allopaths counteract this constipation with cremmafin or lactulose which again are habit forming.

The unfortunate thing many patients do not realise is that sometimes these Proton pump antacids, if taken for a long time, cause achlorohydria (absence of acid in stomach which lead to poor absorption and anaemia).

Homeopathy

Combination A: Asafoetida+carboveg and iris versicola.

Reason

I have chosen this combination on the basis of the principle of "similar treats similar" and all the three remedies have synergistic and common destination for their action.
Combination B: Acid sulph+nux. vom+capsicum+citric acid.

Reason

All these remedies have antiacidic effect based on the principle of "similar treats similar".

I also often advise Isabgol husk which acts as antacid.

Many times pain-killers taken for arthritis or post-operatively are the cause for reflux oesophagitis. Then, in these cases, I have to give them homeo. pain-killers.

HAEMORRHOIDS (Piles)

It is defined as enlarged veins in the walls of anus. It is varicosity (dilated and swollen veins) around the anus. *External* piles are outside the anal sphincter covered with skin.

Internal piles are deep to anal sphincter covered with mucous membrane.

Common causes of Piles are:

1. continuous severe type of constipation.
2. irregular food eating habits.
3. excessive spicy and chilli food.
4. modern allopathic drugs.

Allopathy

Dafflon tablets or local ointments like Proctosedyl or Anovate.

A.C.T.

Effect of Allopathy (medicinal)

These ointments cause temporary relief owing to local anaesthetic effect.

Dafflon causes gastritis in most cases. Systemic or local treatment hardly has any permanent cure for the patient.

Surgical

Most patients feel the result of surgery will be a cure for rest of their life. They are under illusion. I have seen hundreds of patients coming after surgery with immediate and late complications—pain, burning, soreness lasting for many days.

I have seen some patients being given antibiotics for quite a few days post-operatively. These antibiotics cause congestion of anal and rectal veins.

NSAID drugs cause ulceration of mucous membrane of colon, rectum and anus.

Long-term complications like Prolapse of rectum, Stenosis and Stricture are also very common. Relapse after operation is equally common since the basic cause of piles is not removed.

Homeopathy

In my experience, it has never let me down, provided the patient has the will power to control his type of food habits. In **acute** stage following remedies:
Aloe 30 alternate with Acid Nitric 30 + Hamme. 30.
In **chronic** cases with constipation:
Aesculus 30 + Hamme. 30 + Podophyllum 30 with a dose of Sulphur 200 once a week often cures most of the cases. If there is a **fissure** also, which often is, then Collinsonia 30 alternate with Nux Vomica 30 (if loose motions).
If piles is associated with liver infection, which is often the case, then Cardus MQ 5 drops BD after meals works very well.

Case

Chronic Gastritis: A 50-year-old man, Secretary in the Ministry, came with complaint of "Never done feeling" of bowels. He used to feel uncomfortable in epigastrium and pressure feeling in precordial region, air in G.I. intestinal tract seemed to be trapped (incarcerated flatus). His wife told me he has irresistible sleep after meals. Very dry throat. All investigations by Gastroenterologists and Cardiologists could not find anything positive and had advised him Valium which caused depression over a period. Before he came to me, he had Homeopathic treatment from a renowned doctor with some relief but got relapses. I gave him the following treatment and the results were marvellous.

A.C.T.

Homeopathy

Crategus Q + Cactus Q (1:1) BD after meals, Nux Mos 200 at night, Abies Nig 30 TDS along with Kali Phos 6x TDS.

In contrast, **Allopathic** treatment that he had was Ranitidine which used to cause constipation. Ocid also used to cause heaviness of head.

HERNIA

A.C.T.

It is primarily a surgical condition. However, Homeopathy is applicable in two types of cases.
Firstly, in initial stages of Inguinal or Femoral Hernia. Secondly, cases unfit for operation due to any other associated condition or old age.

Homeopathy

Nux Vom in **increasing** dilutions commencing from 200 to 10M alternate with Conium 200.

Case I

I cured one case of a Marine Engineer, 53-year-old, who could not undergo operation since the death of his wife who was operated upon for Haematemesis (bleeding in intestine) which occured due to prolonged intake of combiflam.

Case II

A young boy of 22 years, working under me, had hernia and he could not afford to have treatment. I gave him only Nux Vomica 200 and onwards in increasing dilutions. I did not give him Conium since he was not hypochondriac like the previous one.

Incisional Hernia

Following any abdominal operation one needs only surgical treatment.

HEPATITIS

A.C.T.

The common infective hepatitis transmitted through

infected water, food or drink with incubation period of 20-40 days.

Hepatitis B

Common amongst drug addicts and through infected blood transfusion, has incubation period of 1-6 months.

Allopathy

B Complex, Liv 52, rest and easily digestible food. There is hardly any treatment in Allopathy except the nature takes its own course. Some cases are fatal by going into Acute Hepatitic failure.

Homeopathy

I have treated numerous moderate cases of Hepatitis A with Homeopathic treatment with biluribin level of 13 mg.

1. Sulphur 200 once in morning to start the treatment. From 2nd day Bryonia 30, China 6 and Chelidonium 30 in cyclic order.
2. In **severe** cases, I give Chionanthus Q + Cardus M Q (1:1) 5-8 drops every 2-4 hours. Jaundice due to Quinine and alcohol respond to this treatment.
3. Severe Jaundice in terminal stages of Cancer, prolonged illness, Stomatitis with thrush, tenderness in Epigastrium and hypochondriac respond very well to Hydrastasis 30 alternate with Chionanthus Q.
4. Jaundice of the **new born**: To infants newly born, whose mothers were given hot food and dry fruit, I gave Podo alt with Pulsatilla 6.

ABDOMINAL COLIC

A.C.T.

It is one of the commonest symptoms encountered in children and adults. Firstly, the cause must be found and treated accordingly.

Allopathy

Buscopan, Baralgan, Colimax.

Effect of Allopathy

Constipation, and in old age, prostatic hypertrophy can get aggravated.

Homeopathy

In comparison to the above Magnesium Phos 30 (dilution), Cuprum Met 30 and Colocynth 30 have never let me down.

ANUS ITCHING

Allopathy

It is one of the commonest symptoms in children. After excluding worms as the cause, give a course of Albendazol and if the itching still persists, then the following:

Homeopathy

Cina 200 twice a week and Sulphur 30, 200 once or twice a week is very helpful.

AVERSION TO MILK

It is one of the commonest ailments these days and the sufferers often say, "Milk does not suit me and it gives me diarrhoea."

Allopathy

Abroad, lactose intolerance is considered to be very common. Various lactose-free milks or with certain lactose digestive enzymes are available, which are expensive.

Homeopathy

I have given Natrum Carb 30, 200 which is very helpful in such cases.

LOSS OF APPETITE

A.C.T.

After excluding any underlying pathological condition, if

the loss of appetite is due to inactive liver, then the following treatment is often successful. Amoebiasis must be excluded.

Allopathy

Allopathically, the treatment given is Vitamins or Sorbilin and Liv-52. Except Liv-52, in my experience, other medicines do not improve the function of liver.

Homeopathy

Chelidonium 30 morning and night and Chionanthus Q 5 drops after meals does a miracle in 2 weeks' time.

Case

A young girl from Durgapur came to me. She was 23 years old and could go without feeling the need of water or food for days. She was emaciated and had tried everything in allopathy and all vitamin injections but to no avail. She was given China 30 twice a day and was cured in 2 weeks.

INCREASE IN APPETITE

Allopathy

After excluding any worm infection, the usual advice by allopaths to the patient is to have strong will power but that often does not work.

Homeopathy

It works. Increased appetite, according to homeopathic principle, is due to nervous dyspepsia. Nerves in such cases are activated and make the stomach empty soon. He eats every 30 minutes or 1 hour. Otherwise he feels burning in the stomach.

Case

A doctor from USA has tried everything for his increased appetite including acupuncture. Nothing worked. I had put him on Kali Brom 30, Sepia 30 and Lycopodium 30 in alteration and he was cured of increased appetite within a week.

CHOLESTEROL

A.C.T.

Medical Professionals all over the world try to find drugs which can reduce the blood cholesterol. Until today no drug is discovered **without serious side-effects**.

Allopathy

Lopid (Isobutyric Acid), Lipostat, Questran, Gemifibrozil. The common side-effects of these drugs are danger of excessive bleeding due to vitamin K deficiency, myalgia, headache, constipation, gastrointestinal disturbances, blood dyscrasia and liver dysfunction.

Homeopathy

In contrast, I have given the following treatment to many hypercholesterolemia patients and blood cholesterol has come down to normal with treatment from 6 weeks to 6 months depending upon the severity.

Lycopodium 30 alternating with Cardus m-Q 5 drops after meals. In some cases Bartya Carb or Baryta mur also helps. In cases of hypertension with high cholesterol, B.mur kills two birds with one stone. Other cases respond to ant.crud or puls. 30 each in reducing the cholesterol.

CIRRHOSIS OF LIVER

A.C.T.

In Asia, it used to be the disease of poor people due to amoebic hepatitis or poor diet while in Western countries it is due to alcoholism. Hepatitis B is another cause. Now it is becoming more common all over the world due to toxic and strong drugs being used to treat various ailments. Prevention is the best principle. But in established cases allopathy has nothing to offer except Hepatitis B vaccine which has, no doubt, revolutionised the protection against Hepatitis B.

Allopathy

Sorbilin and Liv-52 may help in a few cases.

Homeopathy

I have used Cardus Mar Q, Chelidonium 6x and Chionanthus Q in alteration with extremely beneficial results. The only side-effect is increased acidity due to these mother tinctures. These side-effects can antidote with carbo-veg.

7

Emotional Diseases

The following chapter is much more exhuastive, elaborate and different in treatment in contrast to what I have mentioned in the last edition of my book.

A. Nervousness, Stress & Anxiety

The symptoms are different according to age and sex.

Children

Common Causes

1. Hereditary
If both the parents are of nervous nature, highly stung, or during pregnancy the mother has been under stress, the child will invariably be nervous in nature.

2. Environmental
Competitive atmosphere with stress of studies leads to nervousness and anxiety.

3. Allopathic Medications
Allopathic medications taken for other ailments. My allopathic colleagues may not agree. Most of the bronchodilators are given for asthma which itself is a creation by allopathic medications, making the incidence of asthma alarmingly high (as explained in my chapter on bronchial asthma).

The common symptoms of nervousness and anxiety in children are sudden rage, certain ticks (involuntary movements of some part of the body) distraction of mind.

In older children, to overcome their nervousness and inferiority complex, they are aggressive, they will be repeatedly looking on one or the other part of the body which is nothing but a replacement of inner conflict of emotions.

Treatment

Allopathy

It has been interesting to note that some parents feel happy when the child is hyperactive, not realising it is due to deriphylline or asthalin, or ventpaed. Often the paediatrician gives some sedation to counteract hyperactiveness.

A.C.T.

Such a child can hardly be expected to be normal in behaviour or in studies. These sedations do not treat the cause of nervousness. These are simply a smokescreen against fire.

Homeopathy

In children: Until the age of 12-13 years. I give them kali brom alternating with anacardium.

In adults: Stress and strain of studies or broken love affairs are the common causes of depression, anxiety.

The other common cause is homesickness amongst students studying far away from their kith and kin.

Allopathy

Often the treatments prescribed are tranquillizers and antidepressants. These drugs do temporarily quieten the mind but the disadvantages of these drugs are:

A.C.T.

1. They cause sedation. As a result, students cannot study properly.

2. They are habit-forming and addictive.
3. Antidepressants cause obesity.

Homeopathy

1. Introspection of their emotions in childhood is very important which can be done only when the child is relaxed.
2. Strictly religious taboos passed on by parents are another common cause for such nervous adults.
3. I find, in my experience, Acid phos, Anacardium and Staph. give marvellous results.

The potency and frequency of dosage depends upon the severity of disease.

Middleage:

A.C.T.

In men, finances and job security, while in women, menopause are the common causes of irritability, depression, nervousness and short temper. The interesting thing is that neither of the sexes knows that the causes of their negative emotions are the ones I have mentioned. They blame each other without knowing the culprit of their negative emotions. They can get release phenomenon if they have insight of their emotions.

Religious insanity, more common in women than in men, gradual and insideous onset without they realise that they have gone partially insane. They feel that they have now direct contact with God. The rituals upset the entire family routine. Such patients also have obsessive compulsive traits and they get upset if they do not take baths repeatedly everytime they pass in front of the temple. If they do not carry their actions, they have the impression that God will be angry with them.

Cases

Children:

A 3-year-old child, a case of bronchial asthma, came to

me for treatment. The mother was very happy that the child stamina is tremendous and does not feel tired. He, however, does not sleep a lot. He has been on bronchodilators which was the cause of his hyperactivity. He was fiddling with everything in my clinic and will not keep quiet for a single minute. His stomach also remained upset due to medications.

Homeopathy

I gave him chamomilla and arsenic alb. He was a different child in 2 days. Then the mother realised that **that is** the normal state of a child.

There are numerous such examples of irritability and nervousness.

Adults:

A 17-year-old boy was preparing for the board exams. He was brilliant but near the exam (3 months before the exam), he became absent-minded and had loss of memory and tremendous confusion.

There was an internal conflict of opposing forces: he has to get admission in IIT but subconsciously there was a fear in case he could not get admission. These opposing forces led to extreme degree of tension which led to depression.

Allopathy

The doctor gave him alprax and prozac which caused sedation and he could not concentrate in studies.

Homeopathy

I gave him Anacardium 200 twice daily for three days.

MENOPAUSAL DEPRESSION

Although there are various symptoms in the menopausal syndrome, these manifest mostly between the ages of 42 and 50 years. Having treated hundreds of such patients, and more and more coming for homeopathy, since the side-effects of hormone treatment are serious and more evidence coming against the use of those hormones. The other symptoms of menopause are dealt with separately. Here I will be dealing with only menopausal depression.

The important thing to note is that many women do not know the symptoms of depression. It comes insideously in the form of irritability, loss of libido, drowsiness, lethargy and loss of interest in day to day activities.

The other interesting thing to note is that their husbands do not know that the change in the behaviour of their wives is due to depression. Many mid-age crises occur due to menopause depression and resulting fight between husband and wife.

Allopathy

1. Tranquillizers like alprax, alzolam.
2. Antidepressants like prozac are the common line of treatment.

A.C.T.

However, one cannot deny the letharginess and increase in weight respectively associated with these preparations, apart from the fact that these are habit forming and do lead to addiction.

Homeopathy

Ignatia and Aurum met. have no parallels in the treatment of menopausal depression. However, at times, I have to give Natrum mur depending upon the case.

Case II

A 49-year-old lady came to me with symptoms of weeping, weakness and sadness, loss of libido and no interest in wearing good clothes or make up. She had lost interest in day to day activities.

Initially, I had put her on Natrum mur 1m followed 2 days later by Ignatia and Aurum met alternating with each other in cyclic rotation. She was 50% better in 2 weeks with no allopathic medicine at all.

A month after her initial treatment, I had put her on Natrum mur 10M which had a magical effect. Two days later, I gave Pulsatilla alternating with Ignatia. I did not go to higher potency of Aurum met owing to her high blood pressure.

In three months of treatment, she is a cheerful person and taking interest in everything. Finally, I finished the treatment with Agnus C and Sepia for one week and there is no more aversion to sex also with Sepia and Agnus.

DEPRESSION DUE TO HOME-SICKNESS

It is becoming increasingly common because youngsters have to go away from home for higher studies or for better career because of poor facilities available in their hometown.

Allopathy

Tranquillisers like Calmpose (Valium), Larpose and Alprax (Alzolam) and Prozac. But these medicines play havoc when prescribed for student since they have to be alert for studies and examinations and these medicines interfere with their alertness.

Homeopathy

Capsicum 30, Ignatia 30 and Acid Phos 30, 200 are best remedies for depression due to home-sickness.

DEPRESSION WITH DULLNESS AND DESPAIR

Allopathy

Prozec; but increase in weight is a big side-effect. Stablon: Gastric upset and memory getting affected.

Homeopathy

1. If it is due to impotency, then Agnus C 30 is given.
2. If it is caused by loss in business, then Aurum Met 200 1M is given.
3. If the patient has lost all hopes, then Anacardium, Kali Phos, Arg n. Ignatia and Acid Phos are prescribed.

I have dealt with hundreds of such cases where patients even after having psychiatric treatment still suffer when they stop the drugs which are mostly habit forming. They come at a stage when they get side-effects of allopathic drugs like increase in weight, disturbed sleep, gastrointestinal disturbance etc.

ANGER

Negative emotions being the common cause of many suicidal and homicidal cases.

Allopathy

Tranquillisers like Alprax, Alzolam are often prescribed.

Effect of Allopathy

The side-effects of these drugs are:

1. These are habit forming.
2. These are hepato and renal toxic.
3. They interfere with alertness.
4. Sudden withdrawal can aggravate the condition.
5. Sometimes it leads to hypotension.

Homeopathy

Chamomilla, Staphy and Aurum Met have often controlled many of my patients' severest cases of bad temper. In children of wild temper, Phosphorus 200 controls the temper like magic.

If the above medications fail, then Cina is very useful.

HYPOCHONDRIASIS (Neuroasthemia)

A.C.T.

Allopathy

Often the treatment is Tryptomer (antidepressant) and tranquillizers like Alprax or Alzolam.

Adverse effects of the above allopathic drugs are:

Glaucoma, postural hypotension, cardiac disturbances, urinary retention, dry mouth, constipation and these are habit forming.

Homeopathy

Acta Racemosa is an excellent remedy for females in general.

Hypochondriasis with Depression and Melancholia:

Afraid of imaginary executioner – rat, mouse, cat, policeman etc.

Case

Miss Jain, 23 years old, who was in severe depression, was very intelligent otherwise. She had been sexually abused since the age of 12 years by her father for almost 10 years. She had been on antidepressants and tranquillizers and had become vegetative lacking confidence, even had no interest in opposite sex. I had put her on Ignatia, Aurum met in increasing potencies, and in six weeks' time, she was a different girl (cheerful, happy, confident, taking sound sleep).

Hypochondriasis due to Sexual Abstinence:

This is very common and I have seen hundreds of religious women in Asian countries taking sex as a bad thing since, according to them, sex is a sin (even with their husbands), if you have to be religious. Such women have all sorts of superstitions. They are often short-tempered.

Allopathy

The usual antidepressants and tranquillizers for such cases are hardly a cure apart from side-effects. Tranquillizers act as a smokescreen and do not remove the cause.

Homeopathy

Conium gives magical results in such cases.

Hypochondriasis due to Masturbation

Such cases have haggard face, dull eyes, trembling hands and cold clammy sweat due to sexual excesses. Staphysagria 30, 200 gives very good results.

Most high school and college students belong to this category. Young housewives whose husbands are away for long periods and if they indulge in masturbation, they become hypochondriac with short temper, irritability. In such cases, I have seen that Staphysagria works like magic.

8

Diseases of Gums, Mouth, Teeth & Tongue

APTHOUS STOMATITIS (MOUTH ULCERS)

This condition is becoming increasingly common owing to new allopathic drugs. Most of the pain-killers and some antibiotics are notorious for its causation. Following are the common causes:

1. Bad orodental hygiene: So the dental cause must be dealt with.
2. Sinus infection: That must be treated before expecting any relief.
3. Increased acidity and peptic ulcer.
4. Pain-killers – NSAID preparations (Non-steroidal).
5. Antibiotics.
6. Diabetics and debilitated old people.
7. Emotional stress.
8. Steroids.

Allopathy

1. The common line of treatment is B-complex with vit. C and locally for pain, zytee or gelora which are nothing but disprin in glycerine.

A.C.T.

In my experience only 50% of the cases show improvement with above treatment.

My line of treatment in such cases is a combination of allopathy and homeopathy as given below:

1. Lactobacillus with B. complex and vitamin C.
2. Folic acid tablets 2-3 times a day.

Homeopathy

1. Merc sol and Borax has never let me down. But if the ulcers are associated with constipation, one should avoid giving merc sol.
2. Acid nitric is excellent in resistant type of cases. Out of many cases, I will only mention the specimen cases:

Case I

A young girl of 22 years with repeated mouth ulcers and constipation and foul smell from mouth and headache. She only responded to Xalibio. 200 because of sinus, and to Natrum mur because of constipation, along with my usual line of treatment of lactobacil and B. Complex. However, the ulcers recurred after 3 months. She is a skiny girl with bad food habits. This time I gave Acid nitric and she responded very quickly.

Acid nitric is also indicated in mouth ulcers due to antibiotics or NSAID drugs.

DENTAL

Trigeminal Neuralgia following Wisdom tooth extraction

Case I

Mrs. D, a business woman, phoned me on Sunday morning that she is having excruciating pain in the ear and left side of the face.

On my questioning her recent past history, she had left upper wisdom tooth extraced, where three dental surgeons had a tough time and kept the mouth open for hours. They had given lots of pain-killers which gave relief as long as she took them. As soon as she stopped them, the pain recurred. Now she had severe gastritis due to pain-killers as well as pain around the ear.

Investigation:

I asked for X-ray tempromandibular joints and cervical spine. It was found that she had severe subluxation of T.M. joint on the side where dental surgeons had a tug of war with her wisdom tooth.

A.C.T.

Homeopathy

1. Combination A:
Mezerium and Plantago major. This is given on the basis of **referred** pain and trigeminal neuralgia.
2. Combination B:
Arnica, Ruta and Rhus tox on the basis of **injury to ligaments** and muscles around the T.M. joint.
3. Combination C:
Antispasmotic (The muscles surrounding the T.M. joint) used to go into spasm at night. My formula for that is: (colocynth+mag. phos+cuprum met).
The patient got relief in 10 days' time.
Now she is coming to me for her menopausal symptoms.

Case II

A renowned homeopathic doctor came to me with cervical submandibular lymphadenitis and he had taken the usual indicated remedies himself like Merc sol and Belladona but no relief.

On my questioning, it was found that he recently had scaling done to the tartar deposit on his teeth.

A.C.T.

I have seen hundreds of cases who are **victims of scaling**. They go to the dentists because of gingivitis which could be due to tartar deposit. The usual symptom of such patients is that there is hypersensitivity to either hot or cold temperature for which they go to the dentist. But what is most disgusting is that after scaling, I have seen the sensitivity of teeth increases for both temperatures (hot and cold). Then these dentists advise toothpastes like sensodyn or thermoseal. These toothpastes are nothing but they anaesthetise the nerves temporarily. By scaling, even after polishing, the nerves are more exposed to temperature changes than before scaling.

Homeopathy

In my experience, my combination of Heckla lava and Plantago major powder is a boon in preventing as well as treating tartar deposit and there is no question of increased sensitivity to hot or cold.

CONCLUSION from this CASE. Always take the aetiology into consideration, not only the symptoms.

GINGIVITIS
(Inflammation of Gums)

Inflammation of gums is caused by plaque that sticks to the base of the teeth.

Allopathy

Dentists usually give Metrogyl preparation on the basis of anaerobic germs causing gingivitis alongwith anti-inflammatory like bruffen or combiflam preparations.

Effect of Allopathy

Hell breaks on the patient with these preparations. They affect stomach, skin and teeth too. Dentists send the patients to E.N.T. surgeon with severe stomatitis with lymph adenitis or gastritis, because of allopathic treatment.

Homeopathy

Merc sol. Staph and Bell has never failed me to cure such cases.

TEETH DEFORMITIES IN CHILDREN

Everybody must have observed that with the increase in the number of orthodontists, the number of children with badly erupting teeth are also increasing.

It is important to know the common causes of deformed teeth which in my opinion are as follows:

1. Diet which is poor in calcium, phosphorus, fluoride and vit. D.
2. Thumb-sucking is another common cause.
3. Mouth breathing due to enlarged adenoids and at times due to marked hypertrophy of tonsils, obstructing the airway at the back of nose also lead to deformity of the teeth.
4. Sinus infection in children also leads to mouth breathing, thus resulting in teeth deformities. In this context, I may mention that most paediatricians and E.N.T. surgeons in **India** have the view that there are no sinus infections in children below the age of five years. This is a misconception since I have aspirated thick pus from sinuses in children below the age of five years and they got tremendous relief after this procedure.

Allopathy

Very enlarged adenoids should be removed where this is the cause of mouth breathing. It is the size of adenoids **relative** to the postnasal space which matters. Many deformed teeth in children can be prevented by carrying out adenoid operation at proper time. It is of no use deciding the operation on the part of parents or surgeon after the age of seven years when the enlarged size has already caused complications like deformed teeth or glu ears.

In India, most people are very reluctant to get this operation done even in grossly enlarged adenoids despite the fact that these are responsible for the symptoms enumerated. The reason often given by the parents for not getting operated upon is "Child is too young". They do not realise that after the age of 7 years, adenoids start regressing in any way.

Homeopathy

In moderately enlarged adenoids, Agraphis nut. 3x or 6 potency is of tremendous benefit. In others, I have given calcarea phos in potencies alternating with agraphis nut. and these respond miraculously.

Regarding thumb-sucking, there is no allopathic treatment to stop this habit.

Psychotherapy to parents and the child alongwith Natrum mur has been successful in 50% of the cases of thumb-sucking. Natrum mur must be given in high potency and in infrequent doses.

Adequate amount of calcium and phosphorus (milk, eggs) should be encouraged.

Allopathy

Taking loads of calcium in the form of Sandos calcium or Ostocalcium, is not advisable since these can lead to kidney stone formation. Moreover, silica is essential for bone and teeth and it is not easy to give silica to children in allopathic form.

Homeopathy

I often give biochem salts which get easily assimilated into the body. The common biochem salts given are Calcarea phos 6x, Calcarea fluor 6x, and Silicea 12x.

Reason for above treatment:

1. based on underlying pathology.
2. based on the causative factor.
3. based on principles of similarity.

PAROTID GLAND DISEASES

Parotitis (inflammation of parotid gland) is becoming very common. Allopaths are responsible for the increase in number of parotid gland diseases, by giving anti-inflammatory drugs to the patient. These allopathic preparations increase the viscosity of saliva and, as a result, there is stagnation of its secretion in salivary ducts which cause parotitis. If prolonged, these may be responsible for parotid tumours as well.

My treatment in parotitis is very unconventional mixture of Homeopathy and Allopathy.

I do give homeopathy on principle of similarity and on the basis of inflammation, I give Bell.30,200 depending upon the cause alongwith Streptopeptidase (kinetofort), an allopathic medicine.

Case

A 75-year-old lady came with parotid tumour which was diagnosed as mixed parotid tumour after biopsy at Mumbai. But since she was unfit for surgery, she came for homeopathic treatment to me.

I put her on Baryta carb and Conium 30 each alternatively. She responded beautifully and later I increased the potency to 200. She is more than 50% better in five weeks' time.

9

Eyes & Vision

STYE

It is one of the most common afflictions and is very troublesome in recurrent cases.

Allopathy

Antibiotics by mouth and application of eye drops locally hardly give a permanent cure. Patient often becomes resistant to these antibiotics and develops fungus infection somewhere else in the body due to overgrowth of harmful bacteria.

Homeopathy

1. Staphy 30 alt puls 30. Cal.fl. 6x.
2. Puls. 30,200.
3. Acid.nit. 30,200.

CONJUNCTIVITIS

It is one of the most common ailments in homeopathy. The underlying cause must be found out.

Foreign body should be excluded. In bacterial infections, use of local antibiotics will do a good job.

However, it is in viral or non-bacterial conjunctivitis and allergic conjunctivitis where homeopathy has a role to play.

(a) Viral Conjunctivitis

Allopathy

Topical eye drops benefit majority of cases.

Homeopathy

Euphrasia, Symphytum, and Ruta are very useful.
Internally in mild to moderate cases: Apis, euphrasia and bell – all in 30, 2-3 times daily in cyclic rotation.
In **severe** cases (threatened Haemorrhage) Arnica 200 and symphytum 3x alternately in addition to the above treatment.

(b) Allergic Conjunctivitis

Like other allergies (asthma, eczema, rhinitis) allergic conjunctivitis is becoming very common.

Allopathy

All antihistamine preparations locally or systemically are simply eyewash. The result is that as long as you take these, symptoms remain in abeyance, but soon after stopping the treatment, the symptoms recur.

(i) Acute allergic conjunctivitis

Homeopathy

Apis 30, Bell 30, Euphrasia 30 in cyclic order.

(ii) Chronic allergic conjunctivitis

Calcarea Fluor 30, Ruta 30 and Symphytum 30.

IRIDOCYCLITIS

It is a serious condition and should be treated as an emergency.

Allopathy

Often steroids with antibiotics for eyes are given. But I have seen patients with relapses and gradually having eyesight affected. The following case illustrates the usefulness of Homeopathic treatment.

Case

A senior lecturer (doctor), an opthalmologist in a teaching hospital, was suffering from recurrent attacks of iridocyclitis and had taken various courses of steroids and antibiotics. After a period of short relief, relapse occurred. On my questioning, she told me that she used to get rheumatic pains and a lot of skin allergy for which she used to take antihistaminics.

Homeopathy

Allopathic treatment for skin allergy led to suppression resulting in iridocyclitis. I gave Thuja 200 one dose and on 3rd day I started with Rhus tox.200, 2-3 times daily. Within ten days she recovered completely. She met me after six months and was absolutely fine.

CYSTS IN EYELIDS

Chlasion is a common occurrence in most people.

Case

A lady, 40 years old, came with cyst in her upper eyelid. She had been operated twice and it has recurred. She also had anal fissure.

Homeopathy

I put her on Nitric acid 30 alt. Baryta carb 30. Finally, I gave 2 doses of Conium 200 at fortnight interval for a permanent cure.

BLINDNESS

Allopaths might scoff at the idea of curing this seemingly incurable condition. Obviously except in certain conditions like cataract, detachment of retina, corneal opacity which are curable surgically, allopathy has nothing to offer in other diseases.

Homeopathy

1. Lycopodium is the head remedy.
2. During pregnancy, if blindness occurs, then Ran bulbosus.
3. Due to paralysis of optic nerve, Borista.
4. Blindness due to haemorrhage, then Gelsemium and Arnica.

Interesting opthalmological cases are mentioned under the heading **'Model Cures'**.

10

Bone Diseases

A.C.T.

There are various orthopaedic conditions where long-term use of pain-killers like NSAID preparations cause gastritis, ulcer and piles despite giving antacids alongwith them. Following are a few common conditions encountered by me.

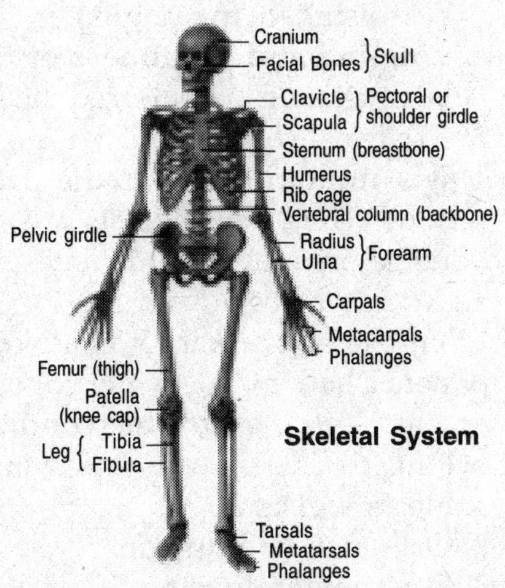

Skeletal System

CERVICAL SPONDYLOSIS

This is one of the commonest conditions affecting both sexes equally. It is becoming more and more common in epidemic proportions owing to modern way of living in the high-tech age. It has become a household diagnosis these days. If the cervical spine X-ray shows some changes, these are often not in proportion to the severity of symptoms of the patient. Computer age has tremendously increased the percentage of people suffering from it. Once the patient's attention is drawn to the bony changes in the spine, then there is fixation of patient's mind on the pathology and a vicious cycle sets in, which further aggravates the symptoms. The element of anxiety and fear gets superaded on pre-existing symptoms.

The common presenting symptoms of the patient with cervical spondylosis are:

1. *Pain: This could be at any of these sites*

a. **Headache** especially the back of head.

b. **Shoulder pain**

c. **Neck pain**

d. **Pain** aroud the ears and the front of chest which can be mistaken for angina.

e. **Tingling and numbness** of finger tips, which again can be mistaken as referred heart pain.

2. *Vertigo ("chakkar")*

This symptom frightens the patient as something is really serious. Then neurologists are consulted who get the MRI done before they exclude any serious condition in the brain.

3. *Nausea & vomiting*

From the above symptomatology, one can know that the patients had to go to the following specialists to exclude any underlying sinister condition. The specialists could belong to any of the following categories :

1. Neurologists.
2. Orthopaedic surgeon.
3. Gastroenterologist.
4. Ear, nose, throat (E.N.T.) surgeon.
5. Psychiatrist because of depression.
6. Cardiologists to exclude any cardiac condition.

Allopathy

After excluding any sinister condition by examination and investigations like MRI, balance and hearing tests, they are put on the following treatment:

1. **Analgesics:** Often NSAID preparations like bruffen, diclofenac, voveran, nimulid etc. These often cause

gastritis and dryness of mouth which may lead to salivary glands infection owing to viscid saliva. Ant-acid preparations for gastritis also lead to dryness of mouth and constipation.

2. **Betahistidine (serc)** stugeron and stametil given for nausea and vomiting are very helpful but cannot be given indefinitely due to their side-effects.
3. **Alprax or ativan** given for noises in the ears that can be habit forming.
4. **To use a low pillow:** This advice does not always work. I have seen that such advice in acid reflux cases could make the reflux worst.
5. **Physiotherapy:** Sometimes traction can aggravate the symptoms.

Homeopathy

Reassurance to the patient

After all investigations are normal, reassurance is very helpful. I had often given the following combinations of homeopathy to hundreds of patients with very gratifying results.

Combination A: Cimcifuga, Causticum and Calcarea fluor.

Reason

All the three remedies have synergistic action on the spinal nerves, muscles, ligaments. As a result, I have found that patients benefit much more with this combination than with individual remedy.

Combination B: Cocculus, Lac Deflon, Gelsemium.

Reason

All the three have action on the cerebrospinal complex, and complementary to each other's action for controlling the balance and vomiting centre.

The potencies of different remedies in these combinations are decided according to X-ray picture, emotional state of the patient, severity and duration of the disease.

Case

It is one of the thousand cases of Cervical Spondylosis I have treated. 50-year-old Margaret Turner complained of heaviness of head, pain behind the ears and, at times, vertigo and shoulder pain. She also had frequency of urination, sometimes uncontrollable.

The following homeopathic treatment did an excellent job:

1. Causticum 30, Rhus tox 30 and Gelsemium 30 in cyclic rotation keeping interval of 2-3 hours.
2. Biochem Calcarea fluor. 6x and Calcarea Phos 6x, 4 pills of each, three times a day cured the patient in two weeks' time.

In **severe** cases, especially in women, I got miraculous results with Cimcifuga 200, Causticum 200 and Gelsemium 200 keeping interval of 3-4 hours between them. However, thin pillow and neck exercises are a must in some cases where I had to give Ruta 30,200.

Cervical rib, which may cause similar symptoms, must be excluded.

GOUTY ARTHRITIS OR OSTEOARTHRITIS

A.C.T.

Unless very advanced, homeopathy gives good results.

Allopathy

Most allopathic preparations are Xyloric (Colchicin) which cause gastric complications and mouth ulcers.

Case

A 58-year-old retired armyman had typical gout with marked swelling at left big toe and has been taking allopathic medicines like Colchicin, Indocid and Diclogesic for the last 10-15 years. When he came to me he had gastric ulcer, still getting attacks of pain in big toe and ankle joints. He was a confirmed case of gout with blood uric acid of 13 mg.

He also mentioned that he gets skin rash whenever he takes xyloric and colchicin (allopathy) preparations.

Homeopathy

Colchicum 30 alternate with Benzoic Acid 30,200, 2-3 times a day as a routine are given.

During the acute attack when there was acute pain, swelling and the joint was hot, I advised Bryonia 30, Rhus tox 30 and Apis 30 in rotation. There was 30% progress in 3 weeks. Then the progress was slow. I gave Medorrhanium, 1M and no medicine that day. Two days after Medorrhanium, I repeated Colchicum and Acid Benzoic. Then he was 85% better in one week. Again, I gave Medorrhanium 10M and started on Colchicum 200 and Benzoic Acid 200 each once a day for one week and he was 90% cured and that was the first winter he passed comfortably after 15 years of taking pain-killers, without any allopathic medicines.

KNEE ARTHRITIS

Case I

Mrs. K, 60 years old, came to me with severe degree of knee arthritis. She is a principal of a private school and does involve moving around. She had knee replacement of one knee in USA six months ago, and is very disappointed with result. She had taken all sorts of pain-killers which give only temporary relief and were causing side-effects. She had used all the modern electrical gadgets available in USA, for knee pain but without any relief.

Homeopathy

I had put her on the following combinations: She had high uric acid.

1. Colchicum+Benzoic acid+Cal. fl. alternating with:
2. Arnica+Bryonia+Apis.

Reason

Colchicum and acid benzoic are par excellence in bringing down uric acid.

Arnica, apis and bryonia are the best combination as anti-inflammatory remedies and can be compared with voveran, rafecox.b preparations without the side-effects of increase in weight and gastritis. Berberis is the head remedy for bringing down uric acid.

She had 50% relief in the first week. After first week I put her on Berberis-Q 5-8 drops twice daily after meals. She has been much better and uric acid had come down with the above treatment.

RHEUMATOID ARTHRITIS

This is the most challenging condition encountered all over the world. Although glucasomine supplement has helped in large number of cases but not in rheumatoid arthritis.

Allopathy

The common treatment given for such cases by so to say experts whether they are called rheumatologists or immune diseases specialists, is – Quinine, Aspirin and steroids.

I have seen innumerable cases in India and abroad, with complications because of the use of above mentioned allopathic drugs. The following are the common complications I have come across in patients taking these drugs.

a. **Deafness and noises (tinnitus)** : These are irreversible side-effects and are due to quinine and aspirin.

b. **Partial blindness** due to the effect of quinine on the retina.

Case I

A middle-aged woman, daughter of a minister, had been treated at AIIMS in Delhi and at a reputed hospital in Mumbai for her rheumatoid arthritis. She has three children and she developed this condition soon after the first pregnancy and the arthritis got worst with succeeding pregnancies. She was referred to me by the opthalmologist who was treating her for blindness with laser. She was sent to me because of her tinnitus and deafness.

Homeopathy

In this case I concluded from my experience with so many patients suffering from this ailment, that the ailment has developed because of the adverse effect of vaccine (anti-tetanus in this case) given as a prophylactic during pregnancy. I commenced treatment with Thuja 1M and that was repeated every two weeks. The remaining days I gave her two combinations alternating with each other. The combinations were as follows:

Combination A:

Colchicum, Apis and Belladonna.

Combination B:

Antim tart, Rhus tox and Berberis. Antim tart was given on the basis of vaccination side-effect.

Berberis was given to encourage the excretion of uric acid products from the body.

It took me three months to bring her condition under control which she could not get in twelve years of allopathic treatment. All that she got with allopathic treatment were the side-effects of quinine, aspirin and steroids, with the basic disease still persisting. After having treated her arthritis, I treated her deafness and tinnitus as follows:

Natrum salicylate and Causticum and Chenopodium. Only 50% improvement in symptoms of deafness and noises could be achieved.

After having controlled the above set of symptoms, I treated her overweightness, due to steroids, partially with:

Apocyn-Q+Aleteris-Q and Gossipium-Q.

Reason

Most of the remedies were given on the basis of 'Similar treats similar'.

BACKACHE AND LUMBAGO

It is one of the commonest ailments these days with sedentary life.

Allopathy

Often Diclogesic, Voveran and other muscle relaxants, traction and bed rest are suggested.

Case I

An orthopaedic surgeon living in Toronto came to me with backache when he got up in the morning. He took Voveran and got severe Angioneurotic oedema and for that he took Avil Retard which controlled the swelling but he was still restless and breathless.

Homeopathy

I gave Cimcifuga 200, Dulcamara 200 and Magnesium Phos 200 in cyclic order with 2 hours interval between them on 1st day and 4 hours on 2nd day. In three days' time, he was cured.

Case II

A doctor, who was very busy in his practice, and could not afford to be off work, was diagnosed as Prolapse Intervertebral Disc by an orthopaedic surgeon. He had numbness and tingling in the legs with stiffness of the muscles of the back. Airconditioning and dampness aggravated it.

Homeopathy

Hypericum 200 alternating with Rhus tox 200 cured the doctor in 10 days. Biochem. Mag Phos 6x and Kali Phos 6x was also given 3-4 times a day.

Backache After Injury

A 45-year-old man came to me with spinal injury after falling from a ladder. The injury involved ligaments, periosteum and muscles around the vertebral joint.

Allopathy

The modern pain-killers help for a few hours but the pain comes back again once the effect of the pain-killers worns off.

Homeopathy

Arnica 200 in the morning.
Ruta 30 + Rhus tox 30, 2-3 times during the day.
Symphytum 200 at night. In 10 days, the patient was back to work.

Backache After Spinal Injection

A 24-year-old lady came with severe backache since she had spinal anaesthesia for her delivery.

Allopathy

She was given Combiflam (Bruffen + Paracetamol) to which she got a very bad reaction in the form of mouth ulcers and asthmatic attacks.

Homeopathy

Thuja 200 alternating with Natrum Sulph 200. One dose of each in a week keeping interval of 2-3 days between them. In between the above two remedies, Ant. Tart 30, 2-3 times a day was given.

In one week, the young lady could do all the kitchen work and look after her young baby without any problem.

Bachache with Leucorrhoea

This unfortunate 35-year-old patient had the above symptoms with foul smelling leucorrhoea, extreme debility and scanty menses.

Allopathy

Gynae-Obstetricians, one after the other, made a mess of her illness by giving:

1. Clotrimazole and Nazral, and antifungal preparations.
2. Voveran forte preparations.
3. D & C which excluded any malignant conditions.

A.C.T.

With the above treatment the patient used to get temporary relief but it recurred in 2 weeks after stopping the medicine. The disease being persistent, she got the following adverse effects due to allopathic treatment.

1. Haemorrhoids, 2. Gastritis. 3. Gain in weight due to fluid retention.

Homeopathy

To this woman with this character of discharge, I gave the following treatments:

1. Pulsatilla 200 1M (morning).
2. Sepia 200 (noon).
3. Kali biochem 200 (night).
4. Berberis Q (5-8 drops) after meals.

In two weeks' time, she was O.K. from all symptoms except some weakness for which I gave China 30 alternating with Carbo Veg 30 for 2 weeks and patient was ever so grateful and cheerful.

Backache with Ankylosing Spondylosis

This is a challenging condition for which orthopaedics and so to say rheumatologists give a grim picture as far as treatment or prognosis is concerned. As a result, patient gets superadded anxiety and tension, thus further aggravating the condition.

In this condition, there is stiffness of bones due to their fixation, fusion and swelling of one or more vertebra. Such patients find much restriction in bending as well as have pain on bending.

Laboratory reports of this patient at AIIMS and other reputed private laboratories were contradictory, but what the patient was concerned with was relief.

Case

A young, 26-year-old school teacher came to me with C. Spondylosis and Sciatica pain saying, "I know you cannot cure me since I have been told by orthopaedics and rheumatologists that it is incurable, but can you give me any homeopathic pain-killers since allopathic pain-killers cause a lot of side-effects."

Homeopathy

I gave the following treatment and she was cured in 4 weeks.

Thiosinaminum 200, Calcarea Phos 200, both twice a day alternating with each other.

Bio Kali Mur 12x and Silicea 12x (4 pills each, 3 times a day). Thuja 1M once in a fortnight.

COCCYDYNIA OR COCCYXALGIA

Pain in the region of coccyx (tail bone) due to:
1. stiffness of muscles and ligaments in old age.
2. injury to coccyx (delivery or otherwise).
3. inflammatory infection of coccyx.

Allopathy

Often the NSAID preparation like Diclofenac or Picroxin or Nirnuselide. Most of these preparations cause severe gastritis or blood dyscrasia (destruction of blood cells).

Homeopathy

In severe cases, where the pain is worst when movement starts:
1. Bryonia 30 alternate with Rhus tox 30.
2. If it had been due to fall, then Arnica 200 alt. with Ruta 200 for 3 consecutive days.
3. If restless and uneasy feeling in lower limbs with stiffness of muscles at achillies calves and coccyx, then Cimcifuga 30 alternate with Biochem No. 19.

Case

A close relation of mine used to have cervical spondylosis and low backache. She is about 50 years old. She used to take pain-killers but that used to give temporary relief.

X-ray showed shortening of space between L5 and S1 and severe osteoarthritis of left knee joint with pain, tenderness, difficulty to stand and even during walking.

Allopathy

Various pain-killers like Diclofenac and Piroxicam preparations failed to give relief except causing severe gastritis despite giving antacid preparations. The patient did not believe in Homeopathy but reluctantly agreed to take when the toxic effects of allopathy became evident. Ostocalcium and Alphodal (calcium and vitamin D) caused gastritis.

Homeopathy

Arnica 200 in morning and Cimcifuga 200 at night. During the day between the above two remedies, I gave Ruta 30, Argentum Mettalicum 30, Bryonia 30 in cyclic rotation at 2 hours' interval. Calcarea Phos 6x 4 pills a day and plenty of sunshine.

GANGLION

Every surgeon must have the experience of the challenge of recurrence of Ganglion after excision whichever part of the body it may be. The usual sight is the back of wrist.

Allopathy

Excision of the ganglion.

Homeopathy

Benzoic Acid and Ruta in high potencies often are successful in curing the ganglion rather than only treating.

FROZEN SHOULDER

This is a condition becoming increasingly common owing to sedentary life style. All the modern-day automatic machines are partly responsible for leading the people to have a restful life and not using the joints for day to day work. Recently, I had quite a few patients with this ailment, almost all had number of steroid injections locally into the joints with recurrences.

The underlying aetiology is stiffness of ligaments and in advance cases, fibrosis of the ligaments and muscles either because of injury or non-use of the shoulder.

Since the advent of computer, I have seen lot of computer professionals victimised to this ailment.

Allopathy

A.C.T.

1. The first line of treatment is to give pain-killers. But in course of time, I have seen that these pain-killers including the modern cox-b inhibitors start causing their side-effects such as gastritis and dryness of mouth. The side-effect of cox-b inhibitors are increase in weight and at times increased high blood pressure and cardiac and brain storkes.
2. After these fail, then the patients are subjected to local injection of steroid, which even a layman knows that it is a temporary relief, apart from bad long-term side-effects due to steroids.

Homeopathy

It may appear strange to an allopath. Even in the beginning, I also laughed that how homeopathic treatment for right and left shoulder joint is different.

In post-injury cases, I find that Arnica 1M works wonders, followed by Ruta and Cal. fluor.

With my experience repetition of high potency of arnica has a deleterious effect.

This applies to both the joints, whether it is right or left.

Case I

Mrs. M, a 50-year-old lady, got frozen shoulder while on holiday trip to Australia. They did all whatever they could, but stiffness and pain still persisted. On her return to India, I had put on the above treatment. In addition, I gave Mag. carb 200. She had 80% relief in the first week but still some nagging pain persisted. I gave treatment for her cervical spondylosis also (cimcifuga and causticum). She is symptom-free now for the last six months despite winter season.

Reasons

1. Arnica for generalised trauma to shoulder structures.
2. Ruta for ligament injuries.
3. Cal. fluor for fibrosis of muscles + ligaments.

11

Accidents

HEAD INJURY

Allopathy

Often NSAID preparations like Voveran, Combiflam, Diclofenol are given.

Effect of Allopathy

Side-effects of these drugs are disastrous if used for a longer period. I have already gone in depth about their side-effects (diseases caused by doctors). If the patient gets an allergic reaction to the drug in addition to head injury, it is a catastrophe. I have treated many cases of the following types with Homeopathy with full satisfaction.

Homeopathy

Arnica 1M immediately, followed on the next day by Arnica 200 TDS. Patients who had the clot on CT Scan and who had refused Craniotomy (opening of skull) and were allergic to most of NSAID drugs were given Arnica. The clot disappeared in 72 hours. In India, this Arnica is a boon where there are hardly any facilities for CT or MRI except in metropolitan cities. Moreover, these diagnostic facilities are out of the reach of common man due to financial constraints.

Case

An Austrian lady, whose husband was posted in Delhi, came to me with history of having had head injury 8 years ago when she fell from a horse.

Allopathy

She had Tinnitus and deafness in left ear since then. She was advised Tinnitus Masker. The treatment was found to be worse than the disease itself; so she discarded the medicine.

Homeopathy

I put this patient on Arnica 200 on 1st day, Nat Sulph 200 on 2nd day and Kali Phos 200 on 3rd day. For three weeks, this was given in cyclic order and the patient was 70% better when she left for Austria. I keep getting X-mas cards every year for the last 4 years and she is extremely grateful to me and completely free from the symptoms.

HAEMOTYMPANUM
(Blood in the middle ear)

Allopathy

On long treatment with Aspirin after by-pass or even having medical treatment for cerebral and cardiac diseases, patients get gastritis due to taking many drugs. Anti-inflammatory drugs and anticoagulant drugs are dangerous in their side-effects. Steroids is sometimes used as anti-inflammatory drug in heavy doses in head injury and in other oedematous sites.

HAEMORRHAGE IN EYES

After being examined by an opthalmologist, the treatment with homeopathy is very satisfactory, whatever is the site of bleeding in the eyeball. In contrast, allopathic treatment can have its own side-effects.

Recurrences can occur even after laser as it happened in case of Margaret Thatcher. Out of many cases I treated with homeopathy, I will mention two cases as below:

Case I

A known friend of mine on official business to Sudan, phoned me that he was having bleeding in his eyes, especially in conjunctiva. There was no nearby opthalmologist available. I knew his physician who had put him on aspirin as a prophylactic in angina, which could be the cause.

Homeopathy

I asked him to stop Aspirin and start Arnica, Ruta and Symphytum 30 potency each. He recovered in 72 hours.

Case II

I was on a trip to U.K. when my friend's 12-year-old son got injury in his eye and his eye became very black. He could not take any allopathic medicine since he was allergic to most of them. He reluctantly (he did not believe in homeopathy) took Ruta, Arnica and Symphytum 30 each, and he recovered in 48 hours.

Homeopathy

No allopathic medicine can compete with Arnica as an anti-traumatic. It has the following advantages:

1. **It is pain-relieving in surgical or accidental trauma by treating the cause.**
2. **It dissolves the clot.**
3. **It is antiseptic.**
4. **It is helpful in undetected injury in other parts of the body.**
5. **No Gastrointestinal upset.**
6. **It controls the fear and apprehension often associated**

with surgery or accident. So, no need of giving a tranquilliser which otherwise ought not to be given in head injury.

SPRAIN

A.C.T.

Allopathy

Side-effects of NSAID preparations usually given for these injuries are given below:

There is no permanent cure for knee and ankle injuries even in surgery. I have treated innumerable cases of sprains (as detailed below) with Homeopathy and that too with permanent cure.

Homeopathy

Rhus tox, Ruta and Arnica are indispensable and have never let me down in any closed injuries to joints or muscles. Selection of potency and frequency of repetition are decided by the experience of the Homeopathic physician.

Case

A relation of mine – a doctor by profession – had injury to post-cruciate ligament while dancing. It was neglected and after 9 months' neglecting, it turned into a cyst. Three topmost Orthopaedics, after seeing the MRI and CT Scan, were divided in their opinions.

The orthopaedics in Mumbai advised surgery but the other one in Delhi advised long-term use of NSAID preparation. She did not find any improvement after 2 months' use of NSAID preparation except the development of Gastritis and Piles.

I was away to U.K. for six weeks and in my absence she went to a well-known Homeopath in Delhi who, without understanding the basic pathology, gave very high potency of Pulsatilla (He told me when I phoned from U.K. to a Homeopath doctor).

The cyst remained of the same size with his treatment. By the time I returned from U.K., I found her knee injury the same as before. On the other hand, she had developed multiple boils and urinary infection due to the use of **high potency of Pulsatilla.**

Homeopathy

I gave the following treatment:

Berberis Q alt. with Apis 200. This treatment killed three birds with one stone (knee cyst, boils and urinary infection).

RECURRENT ANKLE SWELLING AFTER FIRST SPRAIN

Case

This is a common injury in sports or otherwise, but it is notorious for relapses and recurrences and I am sure no orthopaedic surgeon, who is honest to the patient, can deny its recurrences. Three recent cases, that had been treated by topmost orthopaedic surgeons, came to me after getting fed up. Even after plaster cast, there was no improvement. This case was of my nephew, and the other was my secretary. In these three recent cases, **Stroncium Carb** has never let me down.

FRACTURES

A.C.T.

Surgery or homeopathy or both are the mainstay of my approach to fractures. I opt for homeopathy or surgery where it is a must, but what disheartens me is the amount of strong allopathic drugs given alongwith the treatment (except essentially some). Antibiotics disorganise the entire system and every organ of the body. So is the case with the use of allopathic drugs over prolonged periods for a particular disease that kills the person by causing other diseases due to adverse or toxic effect of drugs.

Following are the record cases which came to me after prolonged use of allopathic treatment as anti-inflammatory and analgesic drugs:

1. **G.I.T. bleeding** despite giving Ranitidine because of the use of Indocid as pain-killer for osteoarthritis of knee due to football injury.
2. **Aplastic anaemia** due to use of Oxyphenabutazone given for frozen shoulder.
3. **Kidney failure** because of prolonged use of Tegretol for traumatic arthritis of spine.
4. **Anal prolapse** occurring with most of the anti-inflammatory and analgesic drugs.

Homeopathy

Homeopathy is very effective after surgical reduction:

1. Good callous formation.
2. Excellent as pain-reliever without any side-effects.
3. Absorption of Haematoma.
4. As an antibacterial.
5. For prevention of contracture formation.

In poor healing of certain fractures like **Scaphoid (talus)** fractures, **symphytum 30** alternate with Cal Phos 30 both BD at 3 hours' interval between them never fails. Arnica, of course, is a must.

SPINE INJURY

Homeopathy is tailor-made treatment.

In Cocyalgia

It is a result of injury to coccyx (tail bone): Hypericum 200 (not 30) TDS is the remedy of choice with Arnica 1M once a week.

Allopathy

In COMPOUND fracture, often antibiotics are given for a prolonged period, which not only damages the kidney and liver but also may lead to fungus infection.

Homeopathy

Calendula 30 + Hypericum 30, 200 often controls the infection and, at the same time, the pain.

EYE INJURY

Allopathy

Often anti-inflammatory drugs and antibiotics are given locally and systemically.

Effect of Allopathy

Surgery should be done where it is necessary. What pains me is to see the children with black eyes being put on Combiflam and other anti-inflammatory drugs which cause abdominal pain and loss of appetite.

Homeopathy

In contrast to allopathy, the following Homeopathic treatment has never let me down.

Ledum Pal 30, Symphytum 30 and Arnica 200, in cyclic rotation, every 2-3 hours, have made the black eye haematoma disappear magically.

Case

A young charming lady, 30 years old, was referred to by an orthopaedic surgeon because of air gun injury. It was in the right maxillary sinus below the eye leading to black eye.

Allopathy

She was given Diclogesic tablets and she went into Status asthmatic attack due to allergy to Diclogesic.

Homeopathy

Firstly, I treated her asthma with Ars alb 200 and later the black eye with Arnica 200 and symphytum 30.

TREATMENT OF LATE COMPLICATIONS OF INJURY

1. Fibrosis
2. Osteoarthritis
3. Numbness, Paraesthesia and Hyperasthesia
4. Malunion of fracture

These lead to restricted mobility of the region involved with varying degree of pain.

Allopathy

Often pain-killers, physiotherapy, ultrasound, wax bath are the forms of treatment. Except physiotherapy, other pain killers have adverse side-effects (as mentioned earlier).

Homeopathy

I give two types of cocktails depending upon the type of deformity, handicapped condition and pain.

For **fibrosis and contractures:** Calcarea Phos 30, 20 + Gel 30, 200 + 200 Rhus tox 200 and Ruta 200 often help in most of the cases. Biochem Kali Mur 30x 4 pills, 2-3 times, Silicea 12x, 2-3 times a day is also helpful if given along with above homeopathic treatment.

For **Osteoarthritis, painful sensation,** I give Hypericum 30, 200 and Arnica 200 + Thiosinamun Calcarea Fl 200. This cocktail 30, 200, in my experience, has obviated the need of Morphine and Tegretol preparations.

BURN INJURY

Homeopathy gives miraculous results in IMMEDIATE and MILD to MODERATE severity of burns. Severe or advance cases need hospitalisation for replacement of fluids and plastic surgery.

Allopathy

Treatment for burn injuries in most hospitals, except some in Mumbai, is non-existent and is only an eyewash. Chances of getting cross infection are more than the help of fluids and skin grafting.

Case: Myself

Last year, I was on an assignment in a teaching hospital in Bristol (U.K.). I got my finger burnt while cooking. I went to the accident department of the hospital. The Casualty Consultant told me after putting a vaseline dressing that you will get blisters tomorrow. He advised me to take the antibiotics. I did not follow any of his advices since it would incapacitate me for work.

Homeopathy

Unfortunately, I did not have Cantharis with me; so I dissolved some kitchen salt in a spoon of water and put it on the burnt area. With this emergency treatment based on the principle of homeopathy, I did not get blisters, no antiobiotics. Next day, I could carry out full operation list of seven cases.

Normally, Cantharis 30, half hourly, settles the whole affair in a dramatic way.

ABDOMINAL INJURY

After Ultrasound and CT Scan, if there is nothing serious, one can safely give Arnica 30 + Rhus tox 30 and Bellis Peri. 30 at 1-2 hourly interval. Pulse and blood pressure must be monitored.

NOSE INJURY

Allopathy

After surgical treatment, wherever necessary, anti-inflammatory preparations alongwith pain-killers are often given.

Effect of Allopathy

These preparations cause allergic reactions on Gastritis.

Homeopathy

Arnica 200 at 1/2-hour interval, 3 doses, has never let me down. Arnica kills three birds with one stone.

1. It reduces the swelling and absorbs the Haematoma.
2. It is antiseptic and prevents infection of the wound.
3. It acts as Analgesic.

In case of compound fracture of nose, I add Hypericum 30 and Calendula 30 in addition to Arnica.

HAEMATEMISIS (Haemorrhage)

In bleeding due to injury, unless it is a big blood vessel, which needs ligation as an emergency, my antihaemorrhagic cocktail often helps in the control of bleeding.

Allopathy

1. Replacement of fluid loss is a must.
2. Ligation of big blood vessel.
3. Botropase.
4. Ethamsylate (Dicynene or Revici-E.).

Effect of Allopathy

Disseminated intravascular clotting has been reported in many cases. Dicynene is comparatively much safer.

Homeopathy

My cocktail mixtures are often successful unless there is excessive bleeding. In water, Harmmelis Q + Trillium Q +

Millifolum along with Calendula 30 + China 30 + Carbo Veg 30.

HOMEOPATHY IN SURGERY

Before Operation (Pre-operatively)

1. Phosphorus takes away the fear which is common before operation. Phos 200, one dose is sufficient.
2. Unconventionally, one hour after Phos, give mixture of : Arn.200+Calen.30+Hyp.200 – three doses at half-hour interval. It controls the bleeding pain and haematoma. Arnica controls the shock as well.

During Operation

Sometimes due to excessive bleeding, I use Calendula diluted in water, and apply locally. I also give under the tongue Ham.30+Calen. 30 to control bleeding if I am doing the operation under local anaesthesia.

1. I use Ledum P. in certain operations where I suspect any danger of tetanus especially in surgery which involves nerve rich fingers injury.
2. I use Ruta, Arnica and Rhus tox 200 potency combined in operations involving ligaments, muscles.
3. I use Symphytum 30, 200 involving fracture of bones setting.

After Operation (Post-operatively)

Staphy 30,200 is an excellent pain-reliever in all operations involving stretching, like abdominal operations, Episiotomy and Urethral dilatation operations.

Collapse symptoms **after any surgical operation can be controlled with strontium carb.**

Vomitting due to anaesthetic gases can be controlled with Phos.

12

Nervous System

PARKINSONISM

It is becoming increasingly common all over the world. Nobody knows the exact cause. However, certain allopathic medicines used for hypertension (Methyl dopa) and others used as tranquillisers, such as calmpose, ativan, on long-term use, can **cause** this disease (Paralysis agitans).

Its symptoms are usually of rigidity and tremours. Various allopathic treatments for this ailment have their own side-effects.

Homeopathy

Recently, I have tried three remedies in advanced case of Parkinsonism in which patient has lost his voice in progressive stage of this disease.

1. Causticum 200, 1M, 10M at increasing intervals.
2. In between Causticum doses, I gave Ambra and Baryta carb each 200 potency on alternate days.

The patient got 20% relief in three days after Causticum. It will not be out of place to mention that Agaricus did not benefit the patient.

TREMORS

Tremors in old age is very common and in allopathy the medicines given are often tranquillisers (alprax, alzolam, ativan). These medicines have their own side-effects.

Homeopathy

I often give the following remedies and these are very often very helpful:
1. Ambra. 2. Zincum 3. Lollium.t in increasing potency.

LOWER MOTOR NEURONE DISEASE

Case

This is the case of a 55-year-old man who started getting gradual weakness of lower limbs and was seen by a Neurologist at AIIMS where it was diagnosed as viral. His daughter, being a doctor in U.S.A., got him examined and they said they could not do anything about it. One expensive medicine (Ruelik) was prescribed but not of much benefit.

As a last resort, patient came to me for any homeopathic medicine. His higher mental faculties were absolutely O.K. He has been on Isoptin of 300 mg daily for tacchycardia and AIIMS were thinking of S.A. node ablasion.

Homeopathy

I put the patient on increasing doses of Conium for this ascending paralysis. I stopped his isoptin which was the cause of his neuropathy and extreme constipation.
For his tacchycardia, I gave him Cardiac GOLD drops (crategus-Q+cactus-Q+val+ign.)
For his depression, I gave him Aur.met. and he was 80% improved.

13

Diseases Caused by Allopathic Treatment

A.C.T.

This chapter **excludes** the diseases caused by negligence or overdoses or wrong medicine. This chapter includes diseases caused by allopaths or by patients taking these medications on their own. This chapter explains how the diseases are caused while treating one disease.

In contrast, **homeopathy kills many birds** with one stone. While treating one disease in homeopathy, other accompanying diseases or symptoms are also treated. I will discuss about the common diseases.

DISEASES CAUSED WHILE TREATING HEADACHE

A.C.T.

The cause must be found and treated accordingly, if it is due to tension, migrain, sinus, high blood pressure, cervical spondylosis or eye strain.

1. Most often, Combiflam, Flexon, Ibugesic, Bruffen & Paracetamol are prescribed or taken by the patient off and on for long periods on his own. Following are the

diseases caused by NSAID preparations:

a. Gastritis
b. Skin allergy
c. Haemorrhoids (piles)
d. Increase in weight due to retention of fluids

2. Aspirin (Salicylic acid), Saridon, Anacin:
   Used for long periods for headaches or after coronary bypass, it causes the following diseases:

a. Gastritis, Gastric ulcer
b. Constipation
c. Irreversible inner ear deafness
d. Initiates allergic skin reaction
e. Anaphylactic shock, even the patient had been using it earlier without side-effects
f. Haemorrhage

DISEASES CAUSED WHILE TREATING AMENORRHOEA AND MENOPAUSE (Eye Opener for Ladies)

In primary and most common secondary amenorrhoea, almost all Gynae-obstetricians give hormone preparations and the patient feels happy that the periods have started, not realising the long-term side-effects which are as follows:

1. **Increase in weight:** Without exception, it is caused in 95% of cases. The patient then goes to slimming centres for reducing weight, not realising that they are still taking the medicine which is responsible for increase in weight.
2. **Hirsuitism:** (Hair on unwanted portions of the body). Gynae-obstetricians help themselves and the following specialists in getting rich by causing these side-effects unintentionally.

a. Cosmetologists and beauticians: for treating the above conditions.
b. Gym Club owners make their share in treating these overweight women.
c. Pharmaceutical companies in selling hormone preparations.
d. Dermatologists keep themselves busy by doing thermolysis and electrolysis for hirsuitism, hormone induced acne.
e. Endocrinologists get busy to treat Cushing's and other hormone-induced syndromes caused by these gynae-obs.
f. Pathologists (Haematologists) get roaring business by testing various hormones.
g. Physicians and cardiologists: Heart and blood pressure complications created by these hormones. They give Lasix to reduce weight and other antihypertensive preparations which have their own side-effects.
h. Oncologists (Cancer specialists): How many breast and uterine cancers are produced by giving hormones at menopause and postmenopause? Only they can answer if they are truthful to their consciousness. Cancer of prostate caused by testicular preparations given for climateric impotency.
i. Psychiatrists: Many young girls and women become hypochondriac when they put on weight and develop hirsuitism. They get anorexia nervosa and insomnia and are disinterested in their sex life.

Hundreds of such cases came for homeopathic treatment for artificially induced and incurable diseases caused by our specialists and super specialists in various specialities.

DISEASES CAUSED BY TREATING ARTHRITIS WITH ALLOPATHY

This disease of old age is becoming common all over the world. Although many new drugs have come up but the side-effects of these drugs are really devastating. The pitiable thing is that patients are ignorant about the long-term side and toxic effects of these medicines at the time of commencement of treatment. Since it is a chronic disease needing treatment for a long period, unpleasant side-effects are bound to occur. **Following are the side-effects of allopathic antiarthritic medicines (EYE OPENER for ORTHOPAEDICS):**

1. Advil (Iboprufen) in USA, Bruffen, Ibugesic, Flexon are the common remedies used which lead to stomatitis (mouth ulcers).
2. Gastritis, gastric ulcers and some cases go to the stage of cancer and bleeding despite the use of antacids like (Famocid, Zanetac, Ocid, Ranitidine).
3. Diclofenac preparations under various names cause the same side-effects as above drugs.
4. Blood dyscrasia, gastric ulcer, extremely dry mouth with increase in the viscosity of saliva leading to chronic parotitis.
5. Blocked nose due to drying up of nasal secretions and nose bleeding.
6. Some commonly used anti-inflammatory and analgesic preparations like indocid preparations cause havoc to the body's economy. Anaemia, leukopaenia, gastric ulcer, thrombocytopenia are the common serious side-effects and are irreversible.
7. Some use heavy metals like gold, which in the long-term cause kidney damage and are hepatotoxic.
8. Some use steroids (low strength for prolonged periods). The side-effects of steroids, I will mention under its individual heading, since these are being used in almost

any condition of the body to give a temporary quick 'magical' relief.

9. Haemorrhoids (piles) is one of the common complications all over the world. In USA, almost 85% of the population is suffering from haemorrhoids. There it is fashionable to take pain-killers. Most of these pain-killers cause constipation and inflammation of anal and rectal canal, leading to obstinate type of piles, prolapse and, at times, severe haemorrhoidal bleeding.
10. Recently Cox. B inhibitors (Viox) have been banned because many cases of strokes have occured due to its use.

DISEASES CAUSED BY ALLOPATHIC TREATMENT OF A SIMPLE UPPER RESPIRATORY TRACT INFECTION

a. **Vicks** in different forms, **Action 500, Sinex** lead to tremendous degree of dryness of nasal and sinus secretions causing heaviness of forehead and future sinusitis due to retention of sinus secretions and its drying up of chronic sinusitis and its accompanying headache and premature greying of hair are the result of such treatments.

1. Sinusitis, headache, nose blocking are the results of such treatments.
2. Dry cough is another common symptom because of the use of these Decongestants.

b. Antihistaminics from old Avil to modern ones like Loridine, Cetrizine, all have side-effects of causing extreme degree of dryness of nasal and oral mucosa.

This leads to more susceptibility of infections of throat and nose.

1. Frontal headache and nose blocking.
2. Chronic parotitis with calculi are due to increase in viscosity of salivary secretions.
3. Salivary calculi for the same reason.

c. Decongestants like Pseudophedrine which are **Actifed** and preparations like **Eskold** cause extreme dryness, loss of appetite, constipation and heaviness of head.

d. Recently, Phenyl prospanalene, one of the constituents of many anticold medicines, have been banned because this seems to cause strokes. (Action 500, Cetrizen D).

DISEASE CAUSED BY ALLOPATHIC TREATMENT OF ALLERGIC CONDITIONS

This chapter can be divided into **three** headings, namely:

a. Allergic nose
b. Allergic Bronchitis (Bronchial asthma)
c. Allergic skin conditions like Eczema

For most of these conditions we give the following treatment which often had to be given for longer periods since these diseases can only be treated and cannot be cured.

a. Diseases Caused for Treating Allergic Rhinitis with Allopathy

1. **Antihistamines:** Avil, Phenargan, Terfenadine, Stemiz, Loridine, Cetrizine, all, without exception, have a drying effect of nasal, oral and bronchial secretions. This leads to increase in viscosity of the secretions. Thus Ostia of sinuses gets closed leading to headache and sinusitis.

   These **cause** and **do not treat** sinuses as most of the allopaths believe. These antihistamines induced sinusitis predispose the patient for frequent colds and symptoms of nose blocking.
2. **Terfenidine:** One of the antihistamines at times makes changes in ECG and is incompatible with some of the bronchodilators.

b. Diseases Caused or Created for Treating Bronchial Asthma with Allopathy

Bronchodilators such as Theophyline often has to be used for long. The above Xanthine group (Phylocontin, Uniphylline, Deriphylline, Theolong) causes palpitation, loss of appetite due to gastritis. Insomnia and irritability are the common side-effects.

c. Diseases Caused by Allopathy for the Treatment of Allergic Skin Conditions, i.e., Eczema

Most of the preparations in the market are steroid based. These preparations give only temporary magical relief, but eventually lead to atrophy of skin apart from suppression of allergy which cause other deep seated diseases.

d. Diseases Caused by Allopathy for Treating a Simple Case of Hyperacidity, Dyspepsia and Flatulence

1. Antacid and antiflatulent preparations like Roter (in UK), Asilone (UK), Gellusil, Digene, Polycrol Forte Gel are commonly used and available at the counter.

   Constipation, dry mouth are very common side-effects. Chronic constipation leads to haemorrhoids.
2. H2 Blocker like Cimetidine, Ranitidine, Famotidine, Zanetac and Omeprazol (Losec): These are taken by the patients as if eating chocolates. One should be aware of the following adverse effects when used for long (often it is used for long periods). Gynaecosmastia, Hepatitis, Leukopenia are tiredness, myalgia and arthralgia. Interaction with B-blockers and anticoagulants is well known.
3. Antispasmotics like Stelabid: Used for gastric ulcer and dyspepsia, constipation is a very common side-effect and if the constipation persists for a longer period, it can result in haemorrhoids. Dry mouth is another common side-effect.

e. Diseases Caused by Allopathic Treatment of Insomnia

It is a very common malady all over the world.

Commonly used allopathic sleep inducing medicines are the following:

1. **Barbiturates** are still being used by some physicians. Habit forming and dependance is one of the side-effects and hangover and drowsiness interfere with the normal work.
2. **Benzodiazepines Mogadon (in UK) and Hypnotex (in India)** are very commonly used. They also lead to dependence, the dose gets higher and higher and treatment is taken for longer periods. They should be withdrawn gradually. On long-term use, they have depressing effect on respiratory, renal and hepatic functions.
3. **Tranquillisers** as sleep-inducing medicines such as Calmpose (Valium), Larpose (Ativan) are considered to be safe by the common man. Calmpose is notorious for

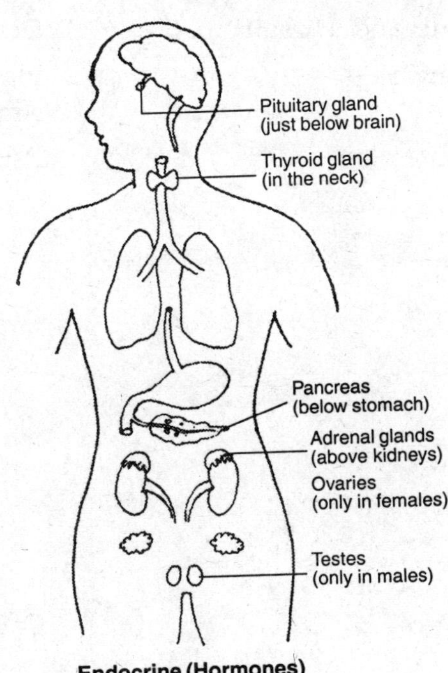

Endocrine (Hormones)

causing depression when used for long periods. Larpose (Ativan) has comparatively less depressing action. When used for years, it does lead to Chorea like symptoms.

Parkinsonism, which is becoming very common in Western countries, is because of excessive and prolonged use of calmpose, ativan and larpose.

f. Steroid Induced Complications

Since steroids are given indiscriminately in every speciality, following complications can arise. These complications make food for different specialists.

a. Gastrointestinal ulcer and bleeding	Gasteroentrologists
b. Hypertension and diabetes	Physicians
c. Kidney problems	Nephrologists
d. Acne and Hirsuitism	Dermatologists
e. Obesity	Plastic surgery & slimming centre
f. Depression	Psychiatrists

14

Heart Diseases (Cardiology)

A.C.T.

It may appear odd and strange to an allopath and they may even scoff at the idea of use of homeopathy in Cardiology.

I will suggest comparative treatment (allopathy vs. homeopathy) in the following diseases.

Now it is recognised all over the world that unhealthy emotions (like Tension, Fear, Anxiety) play a significant role in the following cardiac conditions:

1. Angina.
2. Tacchycardia.
3. Arrythmias
4. Heart attack, if the anxiety is prolonged and extreme.

Often the treatments given by Allopaths are the following:

Allopathy

1. Tranquillisers (Calmpose, Ativan, Alzolam, Alprax, Larpose).
   I have seen that long-term use of these tranquillisers leads to habit formation, Parkinsonism and even depression.
2. Atenolol and other B-blockers.
   Often given to slow down the heart rate but I have seen with this preparation, sometimes the swing goes to the other side, leading to slowing down of the heart rate

and even hypotension. In some cases, it has initiated severe attack of B. asthma.

3. Isoptin.

   Used to be a very popular drug, especially for hypertension and for tacchycardia. I have seen worst case of its side-effects like severe constipation and motor neurone paralysis in a young adult, father of a renowned cardiologist.

Case

I have seen very bad cases of the complications of Isoptin. There was a patient, father of three children, who are doctors in U.S.A., one of them a cardiologist.

Even after reaching the dose of 300 mg of Isoptin per day, his pulse and heart rate were 150 to 160/mt.

His cardiologist son was thinking of Ablasion of S.A. node which again is not without hazard.

This patient was having all the complications like angioneurolic oedema, hypotension leading to paralysis, severe constipation and flushes, all due to Isoptin.

Here, at this stage, (Tacchycardia, Oedema all over the body, BP 100/65, paralysis of all the limbs) they consulted me. My following treatment of homeopathy had brought very dramatic improvement.

Homeopathy

I gradually stopped Isoptin in 2 weeks' time. Gold drops (10 in water), 4-6 times a day. Gold drops contained Crategus Q + Cactus Q + Valerian 3x. Kali Phos. alternate with Abies Nigra 30.

This patient used to get Tacchycardia after meals due to emotional stress. Aconite 200 was advised SOS. In one month's time, his blood pressure, pulse came to normal and stable. Oedema, flushes and constipation disappeared since Isoptin was stopped.

ANGINA

In this chapter, I will refer Angina as to Angina pectoris. Every educated person knows how frightening it is when it first comes. There are various varieties depending upon the type and severity of symptoms. It may be with or without radiating pains.

Allopathy

I strongly recommend, with advances in cardiac surgery, allopathy is the first line of treatment, whether conservative or surgery.

However, in the following paragraphs, I am mentioning certain special types of cases where neither medical nor surgical treatment is suited to the patients as exemplified, with my experience in such cases:

Case I

A 70-year-old lady, a case of congestive heart failure and partial kidney failure and on 15 types of tablets, was having severe attack of angina. She could not tolerate sorbitrate owing to severe headache after taking it. To relieve the headache ensuing from sorbitrate, if she takes aspirin, she gets severe attack of gastric ulcer pain. She already had one episode of haematemsis.

Reluctantly and hesitantly, I gave the following combination to her daughter to give it to her mother. A week later, the daughter came to me to ask for a month's supply, saying her mother cannot live without this combination of homeopathy for angina. The combination was as below:

Arnica+Mag. phos.\Colocynth and Cactus in potency. During the attack a few pills dissolved in water and taking 2 teaspoons of that water every 10 minutes. After the relief is obtained, she could take in the form of pills.

The rationale behind giving this combination (for a lay person or allopath) although homeopaths know as to why I am giving this combination, is as below :

Reasons for the following treatment :

Arnica for fear and to prevent clotting and absorption of clot, if any, occured.

Others relieve the pain by their vasodilator action on blood vessels, so the coronary circulation is maintained. This combination does not give only symptomatic relief but also aetiology based.

HYPERTENSION (High Blood Pressure)

Allopathy

There are numerous drugs and almost all of them have side-effects on prolonged use since most of these drugs had to be used for prolonged periods. Common antihypertensive drugs and their side-effects are:

1. **Methyldopa**: Weight gain, nasal stuffiness, heaviness of head, impotency and Parkinsonism.
2. **Nifedipine, Amlodipine, Verapamil**: Headache, Peripheral oedema, constipation and rashes.
3. **Envas,** Cough, rashes, hypertension, G.I. upset.

In contrast, antihypertension treatment in homeopathy is tailormade according to personality and causative factors in a particular case.

A.C.T.

Mild Hypertension

Crategus Q + Rauwolfia Q + Passiflora Q (1 : 1 : 1), 3-4 times daily as a maintenance dose.

Moderate to Severe Hypertension

Glonoin 2x + Bartya Mur 12x + Viscum alb 12x and Rauwolfia, 2 hourly. The above mixture of mother tinctures is to be alternated with mixture of Kali Phos. 30 + Gelsemium 200 + Coffea 30.

A word for the Homeopath: Most homeopaths base their treatment on the symptoms. Does it mean that if the patient is having high blood pressure but is symptom-free, he needs no treatment? This theory of homeopathy does not hold good in this ailment. Clinical examinations and investigations are a must for such latent cases. So is the case of D. Mellitus who may have no symptom.

Hypertension at menopause with **allopathic** treatment for it, makes a hell of women's emotions and physical strength. These women often complain of other bizarre symptoms due to hormonal changes like dryness of throat, nasal stuffiness, noises in ear, weakness of legs, depression and burning sensations and irritability.

These symptoms get worst with antihypertensive medicines because menopausal symptoms get doubled up owing to side-effects of such medicines.

Hypertension at menopause in most cases is controlled by Lachesis 30 twice a day and then going to Lachesis 200 on alternate nights.

HYPOTENSION (Low Blood Pressure)

Excluding bleeding as the cause where replacement of fluids or blood is a must. However, if blood pressure gets low due to other causes, then in Homeopathy I give Vera.alb, Carbo veg and China in high potencies and as a complementary, Ferrum Phos. 6x tds.

Angina and Myocardial Infarction

Allopathy

Sorbitrates and Aspirin are life-saving drugs, but I have seen in some cases that people cannot tolerate the headache due to Sorbitrate and Gastritis or previous G.I.T. bleeding as a contraindication for aspirin. As a result, in an emergency, if the patient does not have Sorbitrate or Aspirin, then the following homeopathic treatment is given:

Homeopathy

Aconite 30 alt. with Crategus Q + Cactus Q, 10 drops in water repeated (1 : 1) every 15 minutes to half-an-hour increasing interval as the condition improves. Spigelia 200 for left-sided pain and Cactus for extreme anxiety and constriction feeling.

PSEUDOANGINA (under emotional diseases)

This condition is becoming as common as the true angina owing to awareness of the anginal condition. This is more common amongst doctors and health workers or educated class of people.

Since the symptoms of true angina and false angina mimic each other, it is essential for me to give a few points of importance, related to these conditions:

In pseudoangina, which we also label as cardiac neurosis, there is no actual involvement of coronary circulation but due to extraneous causes except due to heart.

However, to rule out true angina from false angina, the opinion of good cardiologist and investigations are a must.

Once the true angina is ruled out, then common causes of pseudoangina are:

1. Emotional (cardiac neurosis).
2. Reflux oesophagitis and increased gastric acidity.
3. Muscular pains especially pectoral muscles (Myalgia).
4. Cervical spondylosis, especially the lower cervical vertebrae.

Allopathy

The treatment is often on the lines of above cause.

A.C.T.

The medications for the above conditions are associated with unpleasant side-effects.

Pain-killers for spondylosis or muscular pains often increase the acidity and cause more acidity and reflux oesophagitis leading to similar symptoms of angina.

Emotional treatment involves tranquillizers which means the patients cannot concentrate and are habit forming.

Homeopathy

The following cases will illustrate the effectiveness and safety of the combinations.

Case I

Mrs. K, a 50-year-old lady, after having been treated by topmost cardiologists in Delhi and abroad, came to me for some homeopathic medicines as she was fed up of taking allopathic for four years.

After all cardiac investigations were normal, I diagnosed as a case of cardiac neurosis.

I put her on the following combinations of remedies:

Combination A: Spigelia+Arnica & Hypricum

Combination B: Asafoetida+Moschus+Abies nigra

Combination C: Colocynth+Mag. phos.

Reason

Combination A is a heart tonic. Spigelia has no parallel. Arnica prevents blood clotting. Hypericum relieves pain associated with it.

Combination B controls symptoms of reflux oesophagitis mimicking heart attack.

Combination C is antispasmotic and indirectly acts as coronary dilator.

The underlying cause for her cardiac neurosis was that her husband died a few years ago due to cardiac arrest.

She had relief within a week and continued the medication for two months. She has no more cardiac neurosis, she keeps coming for other minor ailments, otherwise very cheerful and no more panicky attacks which she used to have when she came for the first time to me.

CORONARY BY-PASS COMPLICATIONS

These are two unusual complications which I was confronted to treat with homeopathy after they were frustrated with the side-effects of allopathic medicines which they were given for these complications.

Case I

A 55-year-old lady had undergone coronary by-pass 6 months ago at a reputed hospital in Delhi. She had been cured from the **real** attack of angina since the operation but has been suffering radiating pain in left arm mimicing true anginal attacks. She had all the pain-killers for that and she developed reflux oesophagitis because of pain-killers.

A.C.T.

Although I did not have details of the steps of operation but it was pointing to the fact that her ribs had to be cut during the operation for one or the other reason.

My conclusion was, some nerves of the left brachial plexuses were **stretched** and **damaged** during this procedure, so I gave the following homeopathy treatment:

Homeopathy

I gave her Arnica, Causticum and Hypericum in increasing potencies and she was relieved of the pain, and for her reflux, I gave Asafoetida and Iris versicola because in her case radiating pain was also due to reflux oesophagitis.

Reason for above remedies

These have been based on aetiopathology and symptomatology.

HEART ATTACK

In this grave emergency, immediate treatment in a properly equipped hospital or nursing home under specialists is the right answer.

In the absence of availability of such facilities, which are hardly available in India outside the metropolis, the following treatment should be handy:

Homeopathy

1st week: Arnica 30 alternate with Kali Phos. 30, every 2-3 hours.

2nd week: Lachesis 30 alternate with Baryta Mur 30, every 2-3 hours. Crategus Q + Cactus Q (1 : 1), 10 drops in water tds.

The above treatment is also useful after controlling the emergency period with allopathic treatment. If the patient is unfit for bypass surgery, then also the above treatment holds good. Some patients cannot tolerate the allopathic treatment. In those cases also, this homeopathic treatment can be given.

Principle of action of the homeopathic treatment in case of Myocardial Infarction:

1. These dissolve the clot.
2. Reduce the work of the heart.
3. Increase the coronary circulation.
4. Lower the cholesterol level.

CARDIAC FAILURE (Congestive Heart Failure)

A.C.T.

If the patient goes into C.H.F. (Congestive Heart Failure) with Dyspnoea, Oedema of feet, weak irregular pulse and loss of sleep, the following treatment is often advised:

Allopathy

Digoxin: Although life saving, but in allopathic dosage, it often leads to nausea and, at times, arrythmias. It acts like whipping a tired horse.

Homeopathy

Nux vom, Carbo veg and Crategus.

Lasix: Again life saving but not without risk, since it may cause electrolyte imbalances. This can lead to cardiac arrythmias to compensate loss of K due to Lasix, addition of Pot chlor or any other potassium salts itself can cause gastritis on a pre-existing gastritis.

Homeopathy

Five phos. is better than Potchlor (causes of acidity) preparations which cause severe gastritis.
To protect the liver from these hepatotoxic drugs, Chionanthus-Q and Cardus.m-Q have to be given.

Cardace: Again, though life saving, but its immediate adverse effect could be Hypotension. Long-term adverse effects are on kidney, liver and taste change. Insomnia is one of the side-effects of most of these drugs. As a result, physicians put them on:

Tranquillisers and Sleeping Pills: Despite their claims of natural sleep, there is hardly any natural sleep apart from the fact that long-term use of these drugs causes hepatotoxity. Most of the drugs used in C.H.F. make the patient a moribund creature.

The following are the typical adverse effects of allopathic drugs:

1. Nausea and vomiting.
2. Cramps.
3. Lethargy and tiredness.
4. Irritability.
5. Weakness.

Homeopathy

China and Chelidonium will protect the liver.
Stropanthus will protect the kidney.

Aspirin: It can cause haematemsis and, at times, severe allergic reaction.

Case

In contrast, homeopathy serves the patient much better without side-effects as will be explained in the following case: A 65-year-old man, working in a foreign airline, after taking premature retirement from the army due to angina, got by-pass done by a well-known British Heart Surgeon. Six months after by-pass, angina recurred. He was worse than what he was before the by-pass. He was on Digoxin, Lasix, Calmpose, Deriphylline, Ranitidine, Potchlor by a cardiologist in Sita Ram Bharti Hospital in Delhi. He sought a second opinion and was admitted in a private nursing home where the physician labelled him as Status Asthmatics. He was confused between the two diagnoses.

I had put him on the following homeopathy with the principle of action.

Homeopathy

1. **Digitalis 6:** For weak dilated heart without the side-effects of allopathic Digoxin.
2. **Stropanthus Q:** It is an excellent diuretic without the side-effects of Lasix and Cardace. It increases the systole and diminishes the rapidity. It has no cumulative effects and restores tone to a brittle heart.
3. **Convalaria Q:** It is an excellent heart remedy in decompensated heart where the heart is overdistended and dilatation had begun and where absence of compensatory hypertrophy and venous stasis had been there.
4. **Crategus Q:** It is a heart tonic and can be given in any stage of heart ailment. It is an excellent anti-arrythmic, sedative in irritable patients with cardiac symptoms.

I had put the above case with a cocktail of all the above mixtures and he responded miraculously in all aspects. I stopped his Digoxin, Lasix, Calmpose. Anyhow, if he found slight irregularity in food which disturbed his cardiac rhythm, then Abies nigra 30, three doses at half-hour interval, would solve the problem.

CONGESTIVE HEART FAILURE

Most of the physicians and cardiologists have encountered numerous such cases from time to time, some before coronary by-pass and some after coronary by-pass.

Most of these cases gradually drift into kidney failure as well.

Out of many cases, which I was called to treat, especially when allopathic treatment in such cases has reached to its limitations, I will just mention one of the most advanced cases.

A lady, 74 years old, Mrs. M, who was treated by two cardiologists in Delhi, was having the following signs, symptoms and allopathic treatment before her daughter came to me for her treatment.

1. She had cardiac dyspnoea, could not lie straight.
2. She had extreme weakness, hardly able to move from the bed.
3. Complete loss of appetite.
4. Hardly any sound sleep.
5. She had oedema over the legs and also puffiness of the eyes.
6. She used to get anginal attacks in between.

Allopathy

She was on the following treatment before coming to me:

1. Lasix 40 mg twice daily.
2. Digoxin 5 mg daily.
3. Omeprazole 20 mg daily.
4. Pot klor 1 tablet daily.
5. Diazepam 5 mg daily.
6. Sorbitrate s.o.s., in addition to monotrate (long acting), which she was taking daily.
7. Aspirin 75 mg daily.
8. Lactulose or dulcolax depending upon severity of constipation.

Homeopathy

A.C.T.

Any allopath knows at heart as to how the patient feels on that much of medication, although these are the correct medications, but to counteract the side-effect of one medicine, one has to give the other medicine.

I gave the following homeopathic treatment, which was based on **aetiology** and **symptoms** and **clinical investigations.** Here the homeopaths should realise that symptoms are **modified owing to lot of allopathic medications. So to treat such patients symptomatically alone is getting into bewilderness.**

Reason for giving the follwing remedies:

1. I gave Stropanthus and Apis for her oedema. Since her blood urea was 87 mg and creatinine 7mg, these helped her a lot.
2. For tremendous weakness, I gave her Acid phos, China and Digitalis (6).
3. For her constipation, I gave her Alumina and Ambra. Ambra is excellent for oldage constipation owing to poor peristalsis. Alumina is given because of extreme dryness due to diuretic effect of Lasix.
4. For her anginal attacks, I gave her Arnica+Mag. phos.+Colocynth. (These work like antispasmotic).
5. For her sleep, I gave Valleriana 200+Kali phos. 30, 2-3 times daily. This combination works far better than Ativan, Alprax or Alzolam. Moreover, homeopathy has no side-effects unlike Alprax which is habit forming and, on long-term, causes depression.

As a result of homeopathic treatment, she is more than 50% better, despite the fact that her allopathic medicines have been reduced to very essential ones.

CARDIAC NEUROSIS

This condition literally means that the patient is worried and thinks that he or she is suffering from heart condition while actually he is not. The symptoms mimic of angina or heart attack.

Symptoms of this condition are that the patient has got pain or discomfort in the chest region, with radiating pain to the arm and back of chest or to the neck.

The clinical examination and all the cardiac investigations have ruled out that it is heart condition.

But the patient still keeps worrying that probably the doctor does not tell the truth or the doctor may not be sure about his diagnosis.

The conditions which often give similar symptoms are the following:

1. Reflux oesophagitis with increased hyperacidity.
2. Cervical spondylosis.
3. Muscular pain due to strain of the pectoral or biceps muscle.

The condition is common amongst the doctors, nurses, paramedical staff or people with awareness of the disease.

Allopathy

1. Tranquillizers and reassurance are the line of treatment.
2. If the patients get into depression and fear, then anti-depressants are given alongwith tranquillizers.

A.C.T.

Tranquillizers, like diazepam or prozec, cause their own side-effects apart from being habit forming and putting on weight.

Homeopathy

1. Reassurance after all the cardiac investigations are normal.

2. I give treatment on the lines of conditions, the symptoms of which mimic of angina, reflux oesophagitis, cervical spondylosis and the most important, for underlying anxiety.
   Spigelia, Arnica, Mag phos. combination works in most of the cases.

Reason

This combination is excellent for left side pain, whether true or false angina. It is **coronary dilator, prevents blood clotting and is antispasmotic.**

Cimcifuga, Causticum and Calcarea fl. works in other types of cases.

Reason

This combination works on the **lines of cervical spondylosis.**

Asafoetida, Iris. Vers, Abies nig and Carboveg for reflux oesophagitis symptoms, which mimic angina. These remedies also control the antiperistaltic movements in upper part of intestine.

Reason

All the above remedies prescribed are for upward peristalsis and are complementary in their actions.

In the **worst cases,** where there is sweating and palpitation, cactus and tabacum often solve the problem.

ARRYTHMIAS

Allopathy

All the allopathic drugs in anti-arrythmias have disastrous and potentially dangerous side-effects. Whether it is Verapamil (Isoptin), Quinidine, Lignocain or Betablockers, in brief, these may cause hypotension, Bradycardia,

Neurological symptoms, Angioneurotic oedema, weakness, debility due to Bradycardia.

Homeopathy

My detailed treatment of the following case with homeopathy will illustrate the perils of allopathy and miracles of homeopathy. A 52-year-old man, one of my family friends, came to me with a difficulty in speech as a result of paralysis which was ascending from lower extremities up into the neck. This patient, on my questioning, told me that he has been on Isoptin (Verapamil) for the last 10 years in 250 mg dosage per day for his Arrythmias which was often occurring after meals or due to emotional upset. His two children are cardiologists and were thinking of Ablasion of the S.A. node since at times pulse used to go up to 180/minute. He developed paralysis recently after getting weaker and weaker gradually.

May I ask these cardiac specialists, "Is this the way to treat a disease at the expense of causing another disease?" On my suggestion of homeopathy, his both cardiologist children felt very apprehensive and doubtful if homeopathy would work in cardiology. This patient developed paralysis due to hypotension induced by anti-arrythmic drugs. I cured the patient on three counts and stopped all the allopathic drugs. This patient was on a latest drug from U.S.A. costing 100 US $ a day for paralysis which was hardly doing any good except causing other side-effects. The neurologists in U.S.A. and AIIMS laugh at my idea of treating this Lower Motor Neurone disease with homeopathy which, in my assessment, was caused by cardiologists with these anti-arrythmic drugs. Neurologists gave this patient six months to live.

In two weeks' time, I gradually stopped Verapamil and replaced it with cocktail of:

1. Crategus Q + Cactus + Convalaria Q + Valeriana + Kali Phos. 30.

2. Stropanthus Q + Gel 30 to get rid of his angioneuratic oedema and rashes.
3. Abies Nigra 30, 2-3 times a day for his tachycardia due to meals.
4. Aconite 200 SOS if emotional upset caused palpitation.

He recovered completely from palpitation, arrythmia, rashes (hives) and oedema. His pulse now remains 75-80/minute. No constipation.

In his paralysis, I gave Conium 200 1M, 10M and Causticum 200 1M.

From time to time, Gelsemium 200 when there was apprehension and fear of death.

Due to diuretic action of Verapamil and loss of salts and resulting weakness and cramps, I gave Five Phos 3-4 times a day.

Now, the patient is fit and fine whom the Neurologists at AIIMS and Safdarjung in Delhi and in U.S.A. gave only six months to live. It is three years since I treated him last.

ANTIBIOTICS

A.C.T.

Very often the use of antibiotics is a life-saving treatment but owing to their side-effects or allergic reactions, homeopathic treatment becomes indispensable.

To counter the side-effects of antibiotics with allopathic treatment means creating other complications:

1. The commonest side-effects are: Gastrointestinal disturbances like nausea, vomitting, abdominal pain and diarrhoea or constipation.

Homeopathy Antidote:

These are antidoted by Nux Vomica, Carbo Veg, Mag Phos, China and Nitric acid.

2. Fungal overgrowth, often in groins, armpits and in mouth.

3. Thuja 30 and Lachesis 30 alternating with each other.
4. Haemorrhoids due to antibiotics is very common. Often the physicians advise ointments which are only smokescreen against fire. Allopathic treatments like Anovate or Proctosedyl do not treat the cause of haemorrhoids.
5. Aloe and Nux Vomica and Nitric acid have a magical effect on piles caused by antibiotics.

15

Skin Diseases (Dermatology)

BARBER'S ITCH

It is quite a common condition.

Allopathy

Most people try one or the other antibiotics until after repeated use of antibiotics, resistance develops to the antibiotics.

Homeopathy

Rhus tox 30 and, if this fails, Lachesis 30, 3-4 times a day. In resistant cases with lot of itching, Graphites 30 is very useful.

FINGER SKIN CRACKS

A.C.T.

I have seen hundreds of such cases and I am sorry to say that **not** a single case was cured **permanently** by allopathy.

Allopathy

Most of the allopathic preparations are steroid creams. As long as you use them, it is O.K. When you stop them, it recurs.

Homeopathy

Petroleum in different potencies with Biochem Calcarea Phos 12x and Silicea 12x have cured most of the patients. In **resistant** cases, focus of infection must be removed such as Pyorrhoea, Sinus, bad tonsils.

DANDRUFF

A.C.T.

It is the price of modern civilisation. The fashion of keeping the hair dry by not using coconut, or other non-perfumed oil is one of the common causes of dandruff.

Use of perfumed hair cream or different glossy shampoos is also responsible for dandruff. Advices by dermatologists that the particular person's skin is too dry or too oily, are ridiculous theories. On the principle of these theories, I hardly find any patient got cured permanently.

Use of various hair dyes is another cause of dandruff.

Homeopathy

Avoidance of oily and spicy food is very helpful in treating dandruff.

1. Coconut oil
2. Kali Sulph
3. Thuja
4. Nat mur have never let me down.

Sinus infection or dental infection must be excluded. Acne and otitis externa are the common complications of dandruff and you cannot cure these until you get rid of dandruff.

ALOPECIA (Fall of Hair)

Baldness, patch or whole, is becoming more and more common due to modern style of living. Common causes of this condition, to which allopaths have hardly paid any attention except giving various shampoos and becoming rich by hair transplants, are as follows:

1. Modern stress and strain.
2. Sinus infection and allergic nasal conditions
3. Migrain.
4. Modern broad spectrum antibiotics, even some ayurvedic drugs.
5. Various preservatives in foods.
6. Various sprays for setting the hair.
7. Excessive use of salts and fluorides.
8. Use of strong shampoos.

Homeopathy

This is becoming a very common condition even at a very young age.

The various shampoos, oils, vitamins are just a wastage of time and money.

A.C.T.

Causes

In my experience, the most common causes are:

1. Stress and strain of modern life.
2. Strong shampoos.
3. Strong allopathic drugs, even some of the ayurvedic medicines.
4. In my experience, only in a very few cases, genetic factor is the cause for baldness.
5. Certain oils containing chemicals also cause baldness.
6. Excessive use of salt and fluorides.

Allopathy

As I mentioned earlier that allopathic medicines have hardly any role to cure baldness.

Surgery

It is an expensive procedure which a common man cannot afford.

Homeopathy

In my line of treatment in such cases, taking into consideration the aetiology rather than the symptoms, which is evident in any way, I find that more than 70% of the cases respond very well to homeopathy.

I often give two types of combinations alternating with each other. Any homeopath would know as to the reasons for giving these remedies.

Combination A:

Natrum mur, Acid phos., Kali phos.

Reason

Most cases of baldness are due to stress and hence the above combination.

Combination B:

Kali sulph (if there is dandruff), Jaborandi and Acid fluor.

Reason

Dandruff is usually due to low grade infection in some part of the body or keeping the hair too wet or too dry, leading to dandruff.

The head remedy, without which the above combinations do not work, is THUJA.

The potency is selected according to the case. This is given in infrequent doses.

The above homeopathic combinations can be supplemented with biochem silicea 12x and calcarea phos 6x.

Case

Sad and shocked, a 19-year-old beautiful girl came to me because she lost her hair overnight after getting some herbal spray from a beautician. She was due to be married in two months' time. I gave Selenium, Acid Phos for six weeks when the hair started coming back and had grown almost completely by the time she got married.

Allopaths might say that giving selenium in crude form could be equally effective, but I find this selenium causing lot of gastric irritation, if given in crude form.

HAIR GROWTH (Unwanted)

A.C.T.

Cosmetic surgeons, dermatologists, except treating these patients on commercial lines, either do not know the exact cause or at least do not bother to do any research. Many females are becoming victims of Hirsuitism (hair at unwanted sites of the body).

My personal views based on treating these patients are:

1. **Excessive use of hormones** by Gynae-Obstetricians since more and more young girls are falling victims of irregular periods. Irregularity in periods is NOT always because of hormonal imbalance but because of modern stresses and strains which lead to hormonal imbalance and cause irregularity in periods.
2. The second cause of these unwanted hair is frequent use of **broad spectrum antibiotics** which lead to skin changes and one should not forget that hair is a part and parcel of skin.
3. More and more **vaccinations** for prevention of various diseases like foreign Serum cause disturbance of metabolism in the body and that leads to such unwanted hair on the body.

The foundation of such hair growth is established even in childhood vaccinations.

Allopathy

Electrolysis, thermolysis, bleaching or plucking or waxing are the common lines of treatment.

Effect of Allopathy

Black spots, growth of rough and harsh hair are very temporary in nature. Scarring is another complication.

Homeopathy

Thuja is an excellent remedy. Most homeopaths have failed because each case needs particular potency and frequency of the remedy. In such cases, very often we had to go to Thuja 10M potency.

Oleum Jec 30 potency in summer and 3x three times a day in winter gives very good results in moderate cases. Olium Jec should not be given on the day of Thuja and one day before or after Thuja.

Case

A 30-year-old girl, very good looking but sad and depressed, sought my help for her hair around her nipples. Owing to this condition, she was reluctant to get married. I gave her the following treatment:

Thuja 1M every month and Oleum Jec 3x TDS as she was from cold country (USA), so potency (dilution) of Oleum Jec was not advisable. She was happily married after this condition got cured in six months' time.

PREMATURE GREY HAIR

A.C.T.

It is becoming increasingly common amongst the younger generation and they are blaming the hereditary factor. But I find, in my experience, the blame lies in the nutritional aspect of the hair which occurs due to the following common causes:

1. Metabolic disturbances due to various causes like:
   a. broad spectrum antibiotics.
   b. perfumed hair oils.

c. keeping the hair dry – a fashion these days.
d. shampoos or strong soaps used for the body.
e. hair creams.

The best oil is either coconut, Jaborandi or Arnica.

Allopathy

All other allopathic treatments do no good at all. Most of the dyes are notorious for causing allergic nose or itching eyes. Basically, it was due to using the dye and even black *mehndi* which is often mixed with various synthetic preparations.

With the above precautions and the following treatment, premature greying of hair is arrested.

1. If anxiety, tension, stress are the causative factors—

Homeopathy

Acid Phos + Kali Phos 30.

2. If there is general debility, weakness, lethargy, anaemia, constipation—

Homeopathy

Calc. phos., Nat. mur., Carbo veg., Acid picric. in 30,200 potencies.

3. If it is due to excessive discharges (seminal emissions in men and leucorrhoea in women)—

Homeopathy

China, Lycopodium do a good job in some cases while in others Acid phos. and Selenium give dramatic improvement.

4. If premature greyness of hair is due to eye strain—

Homeopathy

Jaborandi internally and externally "kills two birds with one stone". It improves the eyesight and also stops premature greying of hair.

The treatment for premature greying of hair needs long treatment for at least six months.

WRINKLES ON THE FACE

A.C.T.

It is human nature that nobody wants to look old and though may be aged but would like to appear younger than his age, whether man or woman. There are various factors which can make a person appear older than his age. After excluding physical illness as the cause, following are the common causes leading to an appearance of premature senility.

1. **Emotional causes** such as depression, marital conflict and deprivation of sexual relations or excessive seminal emissions, prolonged leucorrhoea are the common causes.
2. **Sinus infection**, especially chronic, leads to wrinkles **on forehead and face.**
3. **Chronic indigestion** is another cause.

Allopathy

Various vitamin E-enriched creams or facial exercises at beauty parlours are only temporary measures.

I have seen patients at times getting severe allergic reactions to these creams.

Homeopathy

Kali Phos 6x, Anacardium 30 and Lycopodium 30, all the three in rotation, 2-3 times a day. If the wrinkles are due to chronic loss of fluids like Leucorrhoea and seminal emissions, then Acid Phos 30, 200 and Selenium 30, 200 are suggested.

FACIAL BLEMISHES

Young women are becoming very conscious and get

inferiority complex if they develop facial blemishes, especially after pregnancy.

Allopathy

Various cosmetic creams are either too expensive or these may cause allergic reactions. In comparison, I find these blemishes are often hormone-related.

Homeopathy

Act.r is often very successful in treating these cases.

BEARD

Fall of hair of beard is not common, but I have seen a patient coming to me with this complaint after using a strong "imported" after-shave lotion. He tried various Dermatologists but to no avail.

Allopathy

Local antiseptic, antibiotic powders, are, no doubt, of great help, but in my experience, I have found same side-effects.

Homeopathy

Sphingurus has given very good results one or other time. As a complementary, Calendula-Q locally and Calendula 30 internally, Hypericum-Q locally and Hypericum 30 internally are suggested.

LICHEN PLANUS

Every dermatologist knows how resistant is this disease to routine treatment. I have seen hundreds of such cases and in my opinion either emotional or dietary or drug reaction are the causative factors.

Homeopathy

Kali Ars, 30,200 and Ant.crud 6,30 are often very successful.

WARTS

A.C.T.

It is a very common condition and often either due to heredity or due to allergy and I often define it as a trade mark of allergy.

Another common cause of warts is hormonal changes at menopause.

Allopathy

The common mode of treatment is to burn by cautery or by acid or by excision, if the wart is a big one.

Effect of Allopathy

In ninety percent of the cases, the wart recurs apart from the fact that the cause of wart is not removed at all in allopathy. If any allopath says he can cure, he is simply bluffing.

The following cases beautifully demonstrate how frustrating is allopathy in warts and how successful is homeopathy.

Homeopathy

I must mention that allopaths and laypersons think Thuja is the only remedy for all kinds of warts. That is absolutely a misconception.

Case I

The author had a wart over scalp 25 years ago which was operated upon by a renowned surgeon in U.K. It recurrred after 3 years. Then I was in India and it was operated upon by a surgeon in India. No recurrence for ten years but wart appeared at eyelid margin. By then, I knew homeopathy and I wanted to try it on myself. But my family advised against homeopathy since it was very unsightly and it will take long time for homeopathy and I was to go to International Congress in E.N.T. in Florida. So, on my way back, I got it removed by an opthalmic surgeon in Cambridge, under microscope. After removal, it appeared beautiful and my wife told me you should have got it removed earlier. However, six weeks later, it came in a very exhuberant form. Then I treated myself with Nat.mur. 10M (since I am fond of taking excessive salt). Now it has not recurred for the last 10 years.

Case II

A 48-year-old woman with multiple warts on face came to me. She tried allopathy, homeopathy but was fed up with recurrences.

Apart from the hormonal factor in her case, she told me on questioning that she had no control on her urine.

I gave causticum 10M and after 2 weeks she told me that warts are withering away but not completely. I gave another dose of causticum 10M and next day she phoned up to say that she has much burning in urine. However the wart has withered away completely. For her burning mictu-rition (due to high potency of causticum), I gave her cantharis 30, 3-4 times daily for 48 hours and now she is completely cured.

Case III

A German woman diplomat, whose husband was deadly against allopathy as he was the chief executive of a pharmaceutical firm in Germany and knew side-effects of allopathy, came to me for homeopathic treatment of warts on genital region and eyelid margin. She had already taken homeopathy in Germany but to no avail.

I gave one dose of Medorrhanium 1M followed on next day by Acid nitric 200 and Acid fl. 200.

For three years of her stay in India, she had no recurrence.

Acid Nitric was given because wart was at Muco-cutaneous junctures.

GENITAL WARTS

Unlike in allopathy, where the treatment of warts is the same, irrespective of the site of wart formation, in homeopathy the treatment of wart depends upon not only the site but also upon their bleeding and whether they are sessile or pedunculated, itching or not.

Case IV

A 35-year-old lady, who was having treatment for her endometrosis, nasal polpi, severe menorrhagia, had recovered with **Homeopathy**, after hormonal treatment had failed and hysterectomy was the only alternative suggested to her but she did not agree to surgery.

Now she developed a big pedunculated wart at labia majora. Although she had treatment of thuja for her nasal polpi and endometrosis, but this treatment had no incidental benefit to genital wart.

Homeopathy and Reason

I gave her Acid nitric in increasing potency and the wart melted away. Nitric acid was given because site of wart was at the junction of skin and mucous membrane.

CORNS

A.C.T.

It is a very common condition affecting the public all over the world. Allopaths blame the shoes but I do not agree except in some rare cases since people wearing soft shoes are equally affected. Thirty years ago, when Dr. Scholl shoes and corn pads came in U.K., I thought it was the end of trouble for my feet corns. But these recurred again and again. Even the corn treatment is tailor-made in Homeopathy as illustrated in the following case.

Case

Husband and wife, who are my family friends, went on tour to a continent for two weeks and on their return, when I asked them how was the trip, they said **miserable owing to corns**. I gave Ant.crud. 200 one dose alternate days. The husband got magical relief but the wife had no relief and also got constipation with Ant.crud. So I gave to his wife one dose of Thuja 1M followed by nitric acid since she told me on questioning that she had bartholin cyst (at vulvovaginal region) which was removed a few years ago. She got completely cured and had no recurrence for the last five years. Acid Nitric was given because bartholin cyst is at muco-cutaneous juncture.

ACNE

A.C.T.

It is one of the most frustrating diseases affecting both sexes, particularly at adolescence. Various theories have been put forward from hormone changes to spicy and oily food.

Allopathy

The allopaths conveniently blame the hormones and many patients, after spending lot of money on hormone essay tests, find that hormone levels are normal. Others blame dandruff which again they are unable to cure.

I have arrived at the conclusion that the patient is concerned with cure without side-effects and not bombastic theories given to the medical students on the ward round, on the possible causes without any hope of giving permanent cure.

Homeopathy

In homeopathy, treatment is tailor-made.

Case I

A young rich woman, who was fond of eating highly spicy food in restaurants, at least 3 times a week, and had tried all sorts of modern, imported, herbal treatments from various beauty parlours for her acne, got no relief at all. On the basis of her food habits, I gave her Ant.crud. and Puls., both in 30 potency three-four times daily. She got 50% cured. Then I gave her Thuja 1m (because of her very fixed habits) followed on the next day by Cal.p.30, 3 times daily.

Case II

An American lady teacher, 44 years old, came to me with Acne Rosacea, for homeopathic treatment. She had tried every modern treatment in USA but to no avail. I treated her with Aur. mur. and also gave medicine for menopause.

I find in gastric origin of acne Ant.crud.6 potency alongwith biochem cal.sulp.6x is very helpful.

RECURRENT BOILS

Everybody has the experience that repeated antibiotics for recurrent boils are not advisable since they cause their own side-effects and patients develop resistance to these antibiotics in case of need in grave emergency.

Homeopathy

In my experience, Cal.picrata 30 and Morbillinum 30 breaks the vicious cycle of recurrent boils. To prevent recurrence of boils and increasing the resistance, Echinecia-Q 5-8 drops in water 2-3 times daily.

DERMATITIS

It is an acute inflammation of skin due to any external irritation.

Allopathy

Often we give anti-inflammatory drugs and apply steroidal creams. Both these local and systemic medicines have their own side-effects.

Homeopathy

Calendula Q locally and mixture of Calen.30+Hyp.30+ Arn.30 relieve pain, inflammation without any side-effects.

16

Headache

A.C.T.

It is also one of the commonest ailments afflicting mankind. Self-treatment without trying to find the cause of headache makes the matter more complicated both for the patient as well as for the doctor to treat. By the time the patient seeks the advice of the specialists, the adverse effects of pain-killers had already completely disorganised the entire equilibrium of the whole body. After months and years of treatment with **Allopathic pain-killers**, whether by self or by allopathic means, **patient becomes an ideal case for all the following specialists:**

1. **Gastroentrologists:** Since most pain-killers cause chronic Gastritis.
2. **Surgeons:** Haemorrhoids and other complications due to prolonged use of Analgesics.
3. **Haematologists:** Aplastic Anaemia (destruction of blood).
4. **Psychiatrists and Neurologists:** When there is no permanent relief, then the patient thinks there is something wrong in the brain.
5. **Plastic Surgeons:** Increase in weight by modern anti-migrain medicines, not only leads to psychological problems but also plastic surgeons get the opportunity to reduce fat by Liposuction.

6. **Physicians:** Anti-migrain preparations for prolonged use increase the blood pressure and Bronchial asthma.
7. **E.N.T. Surgeons:** By causing dryness of salivary secretions by anti-inflammatory drugs (combiflam, diclomol, bruffen) lead to salivary calculi and also parotitis.

A.C.T.

1. **Gastric complications:** Aspirin, Analgin, Suganril, Combiflam, Flexon, Bruffen, Advil (in U.S.A., Diclofenol, Saridon lead to chronic gastritis and many cases are reported of G.I.T. bleeding. Gastric ulcer is one of the commonest complications. Zanetac or Ranitidine are usually taken as antacid and this leads to constipation and dryness of saliva and chronic Parotitis due to stagnation of salivary secretions. All these preparations (pain-killers) cause inflammation of anal and rectal veins leading to Piles.
2. **Medical complications: Increase in weight** due to retention of fluids owing to preparations like Combiflam, Flexon, Ibugesic; Bronchial asthma; and high blood pressure with preparations like Vasograin.
3. **E.N.T.:** Mouth ulcerations (Stomatitis) is one of the commonest complications.
4. **Cosmetic preparations** like Sibelium lead to increase in weight, although manufacturers claim it is temporary. I find patients develop inferiority complex and psychiatric problems.
5. **Haematological complications:** Strong pain-killers (Analgesic) can lead to destruction of blood and can affect bone marrow, leading to Aplastic Anaemia which is a dreadful condition.

HOMEOPATHY FOR HEADACHE

The treatment for headache in Homeopathy for different reasons is as follows:

1. It is very specific and individual-based.
2. It cures the patient, provided the remedy is selected properly. It depends on one's experience.
   In long standing cases, constitutional remedy had to be given, apart from side-effects of allopathic treatment, which the patient had earlier. He has to be antidoted to previous allopathic treatment.
3. Homeopathy deals with the causative factors of headache. I give below specific treatment for specific types of headache.

A. Tension and Anxiety Headache: This is the common type of headache. Most such patients do not admit that they have deep underlying anxiety.

Kali Phos + Gel 30 + Val 30 alternate with Acid Phos 30. If the patient is a woman, then Cimcifuga 30 all in rotation at 2-3 hours' interval.

B. Gastric or Biliary Headache: Due to excessive production of gastric juice causing a lot of gas, heart burning and there may be half headache.

Carb V. 30 + China 30 + Nux Vom 30 alternate with Lac Def. 200, sometimes Nux Vom 200 had to be given instead of 30 if there is constipation.

C. Eye Strain Headache: 1st week: Onos 30 alternate with Ruta 30. 2nd week: Nat Mur 30 + Calc Phos 6 alt. with Gel 30.

D. Cervical Spondylosis: It is one of the commonest ailments due to sedentary lifestyle.

Caus 30 + Gel 30 + Rhus tox 30 TDS. Kali Phos 6x, three times a day along with it. After some recovery, each of the above dilutions in 200 potency on consecutive days, *e.g.*, 1st day Caus 200, 2nd day Gel 200, 3rd day Rhus tox 200.

E. Menopausal Headache (Climatric Headache) : This is again one of the challenges for the neurologists, gynae-obstetricians and physicians.

If the patient starts getting headache first time at menopause and had been reasonably free from headache except premenstrual headaches, I label it as menopausal headache.

The problem arises when such women are checked for blood pressure and it usually turns out to be on the higher side. With a couple of readings if it is on the higher side, then they label it as mild to moderate hypertension and they start the treatment accordingly.

This menopausal headache must be differentiated from the headache due to essential hypertension.

Menopausal headache is easily amenable to homeopathic treatment, which not only relieves the headache but also the other accompanying symptoms of menopause, such as irritability, depression, loss of sleep and gastric and chest symptoms often associated with it.

I have seen many menopausal women being put on antihypertensive drugs which at times have overshooted the mark, leading to severe hypotension. This cannot occur with homeopathy.

Homeopathy

Lachesis is the queen remedy for menopausal headache. As to what potency, depends upon the severity and type of personality. But it does work.

I usually follow with Ignatia and Aurum met after lachesis.

To complement the above medication, I give five phos 6x as an all-round tonic.

In other cases of climatric headache, the following combination is a miracle.

Cimcifuga 200 (M), Sang. C. 30 + Mag Phos 30 at noon and Lach 200 alternate nights. If the patient is chilly with associated symptoms of constipation and prolapse uterus, then Sepia instead of Lachesis works very well.

F. Low BP, Anaemic or Loss of Vital Fluid Headache: China 30 + Carbo Veg 30 alternate with (A) 1st week: Ferrum for morning, Crategus Q + Cactus (1 : 1) after meals BD. (B) 2nd week: Acid Phos 30 alternate with Vera alb 200 (Nat Mur 6x + Kali Phos 6x) tds. Repeat A and B in cyclic order.

G. Hypertension Headache: Rauwolfia Q + Crategus Q + Passiflora Q (1 : 1 : 1), 8-10 drops tds in water after meals:

a. alternate with Bartya Mur 30 + Glonoine 30 (if flushing vertigo, palpitation, trembling of legs).
b. if with depression, then Aur Met 30.
c. Plumbum Met 30, if secondary hypertension due to kidney disorder.

H. Influenzal Headache: Gel 200, Bry 200, Bell 30 and Sang 200.

I. Headache Due to Liver Derangement: Chelidonium Q, Chionanthus Q, Cardus M Q.

J. Rheumatic Headache: Colchicum 30, Rhus tox 200, Bryonia 200 in cyclic rotation.

K. Menstrual Headache: Cim 30 + Gel 30 + MP 30 + KP 30, QID.

***Note:* Most women take Combiflam or Flexon which cause retention of fluids and increase in weight.**

L. Sun Headache: Lach 30, Glonoin 30, Gel 30, Sang.c 30.

M. Migrainous Headache: Sick or nervous headache often in sensitive type of personalities.
Arg.n 30 alt. with Chio Q + Alfa Q + Ave Q (1 : 1 : 1). If vomitting is severe, then add Lac.DEF.200 alternate with Arg nit 200.

N. Acidic Headache: Iris v. + N. vom 200.

O. Emergency treatment of Headache: Damiana Q + Alf Q (1 : 1 : 1) alt. with Arg.nit 30.

Following cases will demonstrate the ugly aspect of allopathic treatment and miraculous result of Homeopathic treatment.

Case I

A 19-year-old Kashmiri girl came to me with Migrain for the last 7 years before the start of her menses. By the time she came to me, apart from severe headache, she had very severe and adverse effects of Allopathic medicines from Kashmir, AIIMS (Delhi) and PGI (Chandigarh). Her mental and physical condition was made a mess. She was obese due to Sibelium, extremely weak and irritable, drowsy due to tranquillizers.

My following treatment cured her in 2 weeks and for the last 2-3 years, she did not have any more attack, since she keeps coming to me bringing other patients:

1st week: Damiana Q during the attack (8-10 drops in water every 1-2 hours).

2nd week: Lachesis 30 and later 200 cured her completely.

Case II

My conviction is that either **surgery or Homeopathy or both** give permanent cure to a patient. Antibiotics have a tremendous role, provided used judicially.

A British lady, 30 years old, came to me in a London hospital in 1967, referred by an Opthalmologist to exclude Sinus infection as the cause of her headache, although she had been seen before at Royal National, E.N.T. Hospital and operated for Squint at Moorfield Eye Hospital. She was already under psychiatric treatment and had become a nervous wreck. She was on anti-depressants. Her X-ray of Sinuses was almost normal. During those days, there was no CT Scan or MRI.

I was not hopeful of the results but since there was no alternative, it was better to open the frontal sinuses. After I opened it, I found 15 ml of pus gushing out and both the frontal, ethmoidal and sphenoidal sinuses were all as one chamber. Next day, the patient was cheerful with eyes in normal position.

Warning to a Homeopath: A Homeopath should never treat such cases with Silicea since that will mature the infection into abcess and abcess will find its outlet in the line of least resistance and it may open into important organs like brain or eye.

Case III

This is another interesting case which explains that the medicine cannot replace the knife always. They can be complementary to each other.

A young British Brunette, 22 years, came with severe left-sided headache and, at times, nausea feeling. X-ray of Sinuses showed slight haziness of left maxillary sinus. Usual Homeopathic treatment like Spigelia, Kali Bio, Bell did not help. Left sinus washout helped for 3-4 weeks and the pain was back again with more severity. I asked the Neurologist at Cambridge to visit me and she was diagnosed as Migrainous Neuralgia and was advised stronger pain- killers. I opened the frontal Sinus and to my surprise there was a small Osteoma (bony tumour) at the opening of frontonasal duct, but was not visible in the X-ray picture. It was in 1969 when there was no CT Scan or MRI. Since then, this girl (now woman) is absolutely free from pain as I happened to meet her by chance after 25 years as a ward sister in the same ward where she joined as a student and came to me as a patient. Never forget the golden prescription that to cure Migrain cases permanently, Nosodes like Thuja, Sulphur in higher potencies must be given in appropriate cases.

17

Model Cures

ECTOPIC AND MISSING OF HEART BEATS AND ARRYTHMIA

Allopathy

Often the treatment for arrythmia is Ace Inhibitors like Catopril or Verapanel Beta-blockers like metaprotol, inderal. These can be associated with severe side-effects such as hypotension, renal failure, palpitation, cough, hepatic, cardiac and neurological effects.

Case

A 55-year-old man, under treatment of a cardiologist at AIIMS, Delhi, was advised to do ablasion of S.A. node. His heart rate used to shoot up to 160/mt despite taking Isoptin to the dose of 300 mg/day for arrythmia and high blood pressure.

Homeopathy

I put the patient on Crategus Q + Cactus Q (1 : 1) and Anacardium 30 every 4 hourly and the patient never looked back to allopathy. It is two years now that he never suffered from arrythmia or Ectopics, apart from side-effect of severe constipation due to Isoptin.

ABDOMINAL COLIC

Case

A 50-year-old man came with severe abdominal colic with loose motions after **iron** preparations.

Allopathy

He has taken Ciplox with Tiniba, Spasmoproxyvon for spasmolic pain but then he started vomiting. He was then advised Domstal for vomiting and Gramogyl for diarrhoea, but still no relief.

Homeopathy

After ruling out Appendicitis gall stone and renal calculus as the cause for colic pain, I gave combination of Magnesium Phos + Colocynth 30 alternating with Pulsatilla 30 which is specific for diarrhoea due to iron preparations. As an antidote to the side-effect of allopathic treatment symptoms like headache, loss of appetite, metallic taste due to metrogyl, I gave Nux Vomica 30 alternating with Arsenic alb 30 (for skin symptoms). Within 24 hours, the patient was back to work.

INFANTILE COLIC

Case

Allopathy

I have seen numerous infants still suffering after taking Balargan, Colimax. An 18-month-old baby was brought to me with severe colic due to excessive accumulation of wind. Abdomen was distended and floated and baby went on crying. Baby was teething and had diarrhoea. Stools had green colour.

Homeopathy

Chamomilla 30, Magnesia Phos 30, Colocynth 30 did a

miracle in 12 hours. Constipation and headache also disappeared.

CONSTIPATION

Case

A 48-year-old man came to me and gave a challenge if I can cure his constipation. He told me that the topmost Gastroentrologists abroad and at AIIMS had tried their best but for only temporary relief.

Allopathy

Dulcolax, Milk of Magnesia, Cremaffin have failed to give permanent relief. He is a very rich man with sedentary life. All investigations were normal and excluded any sinister condition. The power of intestines turned weak due to excessive use of purgatives. He had frontal headache and white-coated tongue due to constipation.

Homeopathy

Hydrastasis 30 twice a day with Aletris F Q 5-8 drops in water after meals cured him in 4 weeks' time.

CONSTIPATION WITH BLEEDING PILES

Case

Allopathy

A 40-year-old lady came from USA with the above symptoms. She was in the habit of taking Tylenol and Advil (Ibuprofen) for her headaches for years. For constipation, she used to take Cremafin. From time to time, she used to get backache.

Homeopathy

Aes.30, Aloe 30 every 2 hours cured the symptoms completely in three weeks.

STAMMERING

Case

I challenge the Neurologists, Psychiatrists and Speech Therapists that homeopathy has an excellent cure for stammering. Cases of modern severity respond very well to homeopathy.

After ruling out neurological or mechanical cause like tongue tie, if it is emotional or idopathic, then homeopathy is likely to succeed.

(a) An industrialist, 48 years old, came for his son's homeopathic treatment after the allopathic failure in treatment of ear abroad. After a successful treatment of the ear of his son, he asked for the cure of his stammering.

He responded only to 50M potency of Causticum. To maintain the result, he was kept on 200 potency of causticum. For the last 4 years, he did not have any recurrence in stammering.

(b) A young boy was about to join the army but was scared in case he will be rejected because of stammering. He had a tongue tie also which I operated and he was 50% better in stammering. Then I had to put him on Causticum and Stramonium. He responded miraculously and joined the army.

(c) This is a very interesting case of a bureaucrat being involved in meetings with various politicians. The stammering used to get worst in public speakings. He did not respond to usual remedies like Causticum and Hyoscamus.

I noticed that temperamentally he was a highly stung person, sentimental in nature but losing temper on triffles and getting depressed on trivial things.

Homeopathy

To my amazement, he responded beautifully and magically to my prescription of combination based on synergistic action and based on aetiopathology of his emotions.

I gave him Aurum met, Ignatia and Kali phos. He was a different man in four weeks' time. I had to give him in increasing potencies.

VERTIGO AND ACUTE LUMBAGO AND CERVICAL SPONDYLOSIS

Case

A young MP came to me after having had all the allopathic V.I.P. treatments at R.M.L. and A.I.I.M.S. (Delhi) and P.G.I. (Chandigarh) for her above symptoms. She had got MRI, CT Scan, X-ray of skull and blood picture and everything was found normal. The psychiatrist was contemplating to give her E.C.T. (Electric Convulsion Therapy). She was on Tegretal for all the bizarre pain she had.

On my examination, I did not find anything physically wrong. She was unmarried, 35 years old, and hated sex. She was put on Conium 200 on the above basis. She improved 50% with a single dose.

For her sensitive nature and involvement of neuromuscular structure of the back, she was put on Cimcifuga 200 and her reply was that in 10 years, it is the first time she felt normal.

PSEUDO ANGINA

Case

A 50-year-old man came with symptoms of retrosternal and epigastrium discomfort and flatulence and depression in heart region at bed time due to excessive accumulation of wind in stomach. Patient used to get cold sweat on the head and fast palpitation of heart. He was investigated by Cardiologists and Gastroentrologists. All investigations were normal (ECG, Ultrasound of abdomen, Gastroscopy). He was put on Sorbitrate longa cting and zanetac. He did not get much relief.

I put him on the following homeopathic medicines:
1. Abies Nigra 30 4 hourly, alternating with
2. Crategus Q + Cactus Q (1 : 1) after meals.

He is symptom-free and has no problems for the last three years.

EXCESSIVE URINATION

Case

A lady, 50 years old, had excessive urination for almost 15 years. She was a very nervous lady and had urination after every one hour. Drinking of water caused frequent urination. There was urge to drink more water owing to dryness of mouth.

All the investigations for diabetes insipidus, diabetes mellitus and urinary infection (culture) were normal.

The Urologists did all the investigations and they were all normal. No treatment in allopathy like alkacitra helped her.

She became very weak due to loss of minerals and muscular weakness became extreme.

I put her on the following homeopathic treatment which cured her in two weeks' time:

Gelsemium 30 alternate with Ignatia 30 both twice a day. Alfa alfa Q + Avena Q (1 : 1) 8 drops after meals.

VAGINITIS AND VULVITIS

Case

A 13-year-old girl came after 18 months of allopathic treatment for her symptoms of infection in vagina which caused itching, burning, redness and swelling of vaginal wall, clitoris, labia minora, majora. She had burning and painful micturition.

The Gynae-Obst. had put her on Norflox according to culture and sensitivity and local antifungal (Nystatin) and antibacterial (Betadine pessaries) but 2 days after finishing the course the symptoms used to recur. It was almost a case of pelvic cellulitis.

Homeopathically, I put her on Apis M 30 alternate with Belladona 30 for 1st week. Cantharis 30 alternate with Sepia 30 for 2nd week. She was free from all the symptoms. Her mother came to me 2 years after her treatment for her headache and told me that her daughter is completely fit.

CARDIAC NEUROSIS

Case

A 38-year-old young man complained of retrosternal pain all the time and it increases when he thinks of it or lifts heavy weight. Chiefs of Cardiology Departments examined him at AIIMS, Army Hospital, Escorts Heart Institute, Safdarjung and R.M.L. Hospital, all in Delhi. Thalium, Endoscopy, all gave conflicting reports. Coronary dilators (Sorbitrates), Antacids, Ranitidine and Omerprazole preparations, Alzolam, Alprax did not help him.

I put him on Oxalic Acid alternating with Asafoetida and all the symptoms disappeared.

It is nine months now, he has no problem and is absolutely symptom-free.

BREAST DEVELOPMENT

Case

A 32-year-old woman, belonging to an affluent family in UK, came to me after hearing from one of my patients about homeopathic treatment for breast atrophy and plumpness. She had breast augmentation by a plastic surgeon in Geneva but was disappointed by the result. The silicon implant had to be taken out. She was very disappointed more so since her breast became pendulous and deformed after the birth and breast feeding of her two children. Her husband had also become indifferent to her owing to this as she disclosed to me in confidence.

Homeopathy

I gave her Pulsatilla 30 and Bryonia 30 and Belladona 30 in cyclic rotation and she was happy to note that the breast became firm, roundish and smooth and also her periods, which were irregular, became regular. She had spent 20,000 pounds on breast augmentation in Geneva.

BREAST DISAPPEARED DUE TO DEPRESSION

Case

A young girl of 29 years came to me for persistent headache. Examination and history revealed a very frustrated, depressed skinny lady since her unfortunate marriage at the age of 20 years. She was just a skeleton. Allopaths had done all the investigations and made different probable diagnoses like Anorexia Nervosa, T.B. and had put her on all the strong medications but they gave no relief.

Homeopathy

I had put her on Mercurius Cyanatum and she was a different girl in 3 months' time, cheerful with round plump breast.

ATROPHIED BREAST

Case

This is an interesting case of a 17-year-old girl with a flat chest. She got examined in USA and UK and everybody suggested plastic surgery which her parents were not willing to do. She was becoming hypochondriac and introverted and shunning the company of other girls owing to very poor breast. She was a good swimmer as a child but now reluctant to go swimming.

I put her on Iodium 200 and she was a different girl now.

DOUBLE CHIN

Case

A 45-year-old woman had short neck with a double chin. The two chins were separated by a furrow of the size of half inch. She was diagnosed and treated by a plastic surgeon but was unhappy with the results after spending 20,000 pounds at Harley Street.

Homeopathy

I gave her Nux Vomica and she was amazed at the results. She met me five years after my treatment and there was no relapse.

POT BELLY

Case

An 18-year-old girl, very heavy weight, had an enormous belly. She had got the Liposuction by a plastic surgeon, but within six months, she was back to pre-operative condition. She came to me for homeopathic treatment. I gave her Nux Vomica which changed her emotionally and physically.

RESPIRATORY INFECTION IN CHILDREN AND ELDERLY

Case

My niece phoned me from Canada that her 3-year-old daughter was suffering from respiratory infection. All the antibiotics, decongestants and steam inhalation given by allopaths are of no use.

I advised Antim Tart and Kali Bio alternating with each other and she phoned after 48 hours that she had a miraculous result.

These types of cases are very commonly created by allopaths and the above treatment has magical effects in curing such cases.

DENTAL CASES

Case

1. Oroantral Fistula

These cases are of interest to my dental colleagues also. I will mention two cases which I treated homeopathically.

Case I

A lady teacher from Saharanpur was treated by three dental surgeons, one after the other, and by two ENT surgeons. They did root canal treatment, dental extraction and gave loads of antibiotics for two years.

Homeopathy

I cured the patient with following homeopathic treatment—Silicea 1M once a week. No other medicine that day. Rest of the days mixture of Calendula 30+Kalibio 30. Calendula mother tincture was given externally.

Case II

A 65-year-old male from Assam had oroantral fistula. After biopsy taken at Mumbai and Delhi confirmed it is benign, he was referred to me. I operated with a palatal flap but after a few weeks, it failed. Then I operated second time with buccal flap and it again failed. By this time the patient lost confidence in Allopathy and reluctantly I told him we can have a go with Homeopathy. He agreed.

Homeopathy

I gave locally Calendula+Echinechia mother tinctures. Internally I gave Silicea 1M, 10M at two weeks' interval with Calendula 30+Kalibio. 200 daily. He was cured in 6 weeks' time.

DERMATOLOGY

Case

An Italian diplomat came to me after nine months' treatment at Skin Institute and at Moolchand Hospital, in Delhi for extreme itching and red eruptions all over the body after doing fishing in South America. He was given every allopathic medicine available by dermatologists—Steroids, antifungal, antibacterial creams and ointments.

Homeopathy

First I gave Rhus tox, which did not help. Then I gave Ledum pal 30, 200. He responded dramatically. He has marked Rheumatic history also.

NEPHROLOGY

Case

(a) A 23-year-old Kashmiri girl came to me with severe urinary infection with symptoms of burning and frequency of micturition, backache and extreme prostration.

She had four courses of antibiotics according to culture and sensitivity (done at different laboratories) but got no relief. The W.B.C. came to 3000. Urine was still full of pus.

Homeopathy

I gave her Berberis-Q+Equiestrium-Q (10 drops every half hourly) alternating with Cantharis 30 and she started getting relief in 24 hours. I continued the medicines for another 3 weeks with increasing potencies and she was completely cured. Urine culture became clear. W.B.C. and Hb. came to normal.

(b) A renowned physician had T.U.R. prostate operation with laser, but unfortunately he developed secondary infection, for which very strong antibiotics had to be given to control infection. The antibiotics caused severe leucopaenia and thrombocytopaenia. However, he continued to have incontinence despite all this torture and now he went into depression.

Homeopathy

I gave him Populus.T.-Q alongwith Sabal serrulata after controlling his depression with Aurum-met. I gave China and Acid phos both in 30 potency to overcome weakness. Finally, his blood count also came to normal. This physician, before this episode, never believed in homeopathy.

OPTHALMOLOGY

A very interesting case from Orissa was referred from an opthalmologist of India fame, with following symptoms:

Heaviness of forehead, reduced hearing and noises in ears and blurring of vision. At times, severe headache. All symptoms were for the last 10 years, worst for the last 3 years.

Past History: She was given Quinine, Disprin and Steroids 10 years ago by a reputed immunologist at AIIMS for Rheumatoid arthritis which she developed soon after her last child's delivery.

A.C.T.

In my opinion, an immunologist might have given the correct treatment as far as allopathy is concerned, but after I have examined the patient and her audiometry (hearing tests) examination and tests done by an opthalmologist, it leaves no doubt in my mind that all her symptoms were traced back to the allopathic treatment for her rheumatoid arthritis. The depressing thing was that the patient was still having relapses of arthritis after having all the disastrous treatments from allopath from Delhi and medical college in Lucknow.

I feel this type of Allopathy should be avoided which creates more severe disease than the disease for which the treatment was given.

Homeopathy

I gave the following treatment on the principles of homeopathy and it took 4 months before the patient had got relief:

1. Thuja 1M one dose to start with because she had Rheumatoid owing to tetanus vaccine for pregnancy.
2. Chininum.sulph.30,200 rest of the days to counteract the side-effects of Lariago (Quinine).
3. Mag.phos 30 and acid salicylic 30, both twice a day alternating with chininum.sulph 30.

She started getting relief 6 weeks after commencing treatment but treatment was continued for six months.

No medicine was given on the day of Thuja 1M.

PSYCHIATRY

Case

A 34-year-old married young man came to me and told that he tried every medicine from all psychiatrists (stablon, alprax, ativan and electric shocks) but got no relief. His present symptoms were:

(a) Inability to decide; (b) Checking locks again and again, washing hands again and again; (c) Taking bath 3-4 times before prayers, even in winter and saying he is a very religious man; (d) He suffers from depression, weakness and impotency. He thinks it is not good to have sex too often.

Homeopathy

In the beginning, I gave Acid phos and Damiana-Q but that did not make any difference. But then, on the basis of his religious insanity, I gave Lachesis 1M, no other treatment on that day.

Then, from the next day, I gave Staph.200 alternating with Acid phos 200 and he got cured in 3 weeks' time.

Reasons

These remedies were given for the reason that he had guilty feelings due to masturbation.

GYNAE.-OBST.

Case

A 26-year-old British nurse came to me with severe itching of both ears on and off. She was posted in Muscat where she developed this infection. Most E.N.T. surgeons tried various antifungal creams, alongwith anti-allergic tablets internally but the condition used to recur after some time. Then she went to Harley Street E.N.T. surgeon before coming to me. On my questioning, she admitted having vaginal fungal infection also. So I realised the reason of obstinancy coming in the way of her treatment. Unless I treat her vaginal fungal infection first, ear fungus could not be cured.

Homeopathy

I gave her the following treatment :

a. Acid sulph 30 and Thuja 30 alternating with each other twice daily internally.

b. Hydr.Q + Thuja Q + Calendula Q applied externally.

The patient was cured in 1 week's time. She was working in the same hospital in Wales (U.K.) and during my stay for 1 year, she did not have any relapse.

Remember the homeopathy principle: "Treat the patient as a whole."

NEUROLOGY

Case

(a) Migrain

A British lady came with severe right-sided migrain. Her husband was posted in Delhi for 3 years. She had this for the last 10 years and had tried everything in modern treatment available in U.K. but to no avail.

Homeopathy

I gave Sangunaria can. in increasing potencies upto 10M and she got completely cured.

(b) Lower Motor Neurone Disease (post-viral paralysis): This case demonstrates that Homeopathy is far safer and economical as compared to Allopathy, quite expensive, full of adverse effects and palliative in nature. An executive engineer got viral 2-3 times at an interval of 2-3 months. He felt very weak and was diagnosed at AIIMS and in USA as a case of Lower Motor Neurone disease and he was put on Riluzole (Rilutex) – a new drug supposed to work for this disease. He was given six months' life span. Besides the exhuberant cost of Ritulek, he was going downhill.

Homeopathy

With great reluctance, his wife agreed to giving him homeopathy, which I gave as below:

I started with Thuja 1M since he had innumerable vaccinations many a times owing to his travel abroad. Then I gave Lathyrus 30 tds and it helped a little but not much. Then I put him on Causticum 200 because of his suppression of severe allergic symptoms with allopathic anti-allergic drug and his voice was weak. He showed 30% improvement in 10 days and got completely cured in 4 months.

NEPHROTIC SYNDROME & BRONCHIAL ASTHMA

A 5-year-old boy, who had bronchial asthma since the age of 2 years and nephrotic syndrome for the last one year, came to me after having taken the following allopathic medicines:

Allopathy

1. Steroids for bronchial asthma and for nephrotic syndrome.
2. Antibiotic (Floxacine group) for kidney infection.
3. Brochodilators, of deriphylline group orally.
4. Nebulisers (both solbutamol and steroid groups).

The above diagnoses were confirmed and he was being treated at the best institution in Delhi, by a nephrologist and a chest paediatrician. During winter, the attack used to be more severe.

A.C.T.

The child was putting on weight because of steroids, feeling weak, because of loss of proteins in urine due to nephrotic syndrome. He could not play with other children for a longer period owing to becoming breathless, because of asthma.

Homeopathy

1. I started the treatment with Thuja 200.

Reason

1. I often find these children develop bronchial asthma owing to vaccinations.
2. This was followed by Phosphorus 30 and Arsenic alb and Natrum sulph. The child showed tremendous relief in nasobronchial symptoms in one week's time.

Phosphorus par excellence is the head remedy for entire nasobronchial allergy, except in cases of suspected T.B. where it can flare up the condition. Children emotionally hypersensitive, with a long neck and narrow chest, respond splendidly to it.

Arsenic alb for its particular affinity for restlessness with thirst for small quantity of water, never fails in my patients. Natrum sulph is a boon for children asthma, especially if there is accompanying eczema.

Mother told me that it is the first time she did not have to give a nebuliser.

3. Then I started treatment of nephrotic syndrome by giving Mercurious corrosive, Belladonna and Apis. The child showed only 50% improvement in two weeks' time.
4. Then I added Terebinth in addition to the above medication for nephrotic syndrome.

He has completely recovered and all the urine tests are normal.

Terebinth and mercurious were given on the basis of Hanneman's principle.

CONDITIONS CAUSED BY ALLOPATHS

This chapter may be unpalatable to the allopaths but one should be courageous to face the reality. This chapter EXCLUDES diseases caused by sheer negligence. The three basic principles while treating a patient which should be kept in mind are as follows:

1. Drug-induced diseases should not be worse than the disease for which the medicine is given. Drug-induced disease could be due to either adverse side-effects or toxic effects of the drugs because of the need of its prolonged use.
2. Patient must be explained the possible side-effects of the drug when it is prescribed in the present climate of litigations.
3. One should be honest to give the patient the alternative choice of medicine in other branches, if he knows at

heart that his branch of medication may not offer better than homeopathy or ayurveda which is safer and gives a long-lasting cure.

A. TEGRATOL (Carbamazepine)

Admittedly, this is one of the head remedies for epilepsy. Except in major epilepsy, to prescribe for routine neuralgias or minor epilepsy, it will cause more diseases than for the disease for which it has been prescribed. Patients had come to me with the following side-effects due to this medicine.

1. Kidney failure due to its use.
2. Aplastic Anaemia.
3. Psychosis, leading to marital problems.
4. Ulcerative colitis.
5. Arrythmias.

B. VOVERAN, BRUFFEN, FLEXON, IBUGESIC AND DICLOMOL DISCLOCIDE

1. Severe gastrointestinal problems leading to peptic ulcer and G.I. bleeding.
2. Stomatitis.
3. Proctitis and haemorrhoids.
4. Parotiditis due to dryness of mouth secretions.

C. HORMONES

Anabolic hormones like Durabolin or Decadurabolin to energise the individual who is feeling mentally and physically tired.

In males:

Prostatis and enlargement of prostate gland.

Homeopathy: Sabal serrulata Q and selenium.

In females:
Hirsuitism (hair on the face) and obesity.
It is difficult to treat even with homeopathy.

D. DRUG-INDUCED HAEMORRHOIDS

This is a condition due to venous congestion and stasis in the anal canal either due to chronic constipation, spicy food or allopathic drugs. Commonly, allopathic treatment comprises local ointments and dafflon internally in bleeding cases. It is also common during post-operative cases for the above reasons.

Homeopathy

Alos, Nitric Acid and Hammamelis in 30 and later 200 in advanced cases.

E. ASPIRIN — LIFE SAVER OR KILLER

Recently, a panel of researchers in USA said that the available data did not provide strong evidence that the benefits outweighed the side-effect risks.

According to a study conducted on more than 55,000 people, it was claimed that five years of daily aspirin use by people at moderate risk could prevent 14 heart attacks for every 1000 patients treated. **But exposure to aspirin will also cause upto two strokes and 2-4 cases of major gastrointestinal bleeding.**

The experts, therefore, are of the view that while more than 100-year-old drug was still good for people with an attack, it should not be recommended to those with moderate risk.

Author's views:

As an ENT surgeon, I have been dealing with epidemic of nose and ear bleeding, due to aspirin than what has

been reported in various journals. It will be shocking to give the figure of elderly patients dying because of complications as a result of bleeding due to aspirin.

Homeopathy

In unavoidable cases, I have counteracted the side-effects of aspirin with mag. phos and arnica.

18

Sex, Health, Allopathy and Homeopathy

It has been proved recently, as quoted by the following authors, that sex is a necessity for health. According to my observations on many patients, this trio: sleep, food and sex (SFS) is an essential ingredient to sound health. According to Michael Roizen, sex has an antiaging effect. In British Medical Journal, in article *Sex and Death: Are they related?* it has been reported that those having two orgasms a week have half the risk of dying from various causes.

A study in *Psychosomatic Medicine* has found that sexual dissatisfaction is the precursor of heart disease.

Dr. Cynthia Watson, author of "*A guide to aphrodisiacs and sexual pleasures*", says that a healthy sex life and overall health are intrinsically linked. She says, "Sex makes you relax, relieves stress and produces endorphins—the body pain relievers and sex help the immune system function better".

Allopathy

Beyond doubt, I have found smile in lot of people's faces after Viagra drug came in the market, but these preparations have their own limitations and side-effects.

No doubt the "Week-end Pill (Cialis) is far better than Viagra". It has smoother onset, less side-effects, and is longer lasting than Viagra.

Homeopathy

The word used by most homeopaths in their book, "*Sins*", synonymous with sex, is most damaging to the readers and patients.

Homeopathy still has to go a long way to compete allopathy in treatment of impotency. Remedies like lycopodium and agnus. c are of limited value.

Sex, Brain, Memory & Homeopathy

According to a German researcher, Werner Habermehl, sex stimulates the brain and makes people more intelligent. Habermehl said that love-making, besides physically exciting the body, also provides sharper brain. Hence, the increased amount of adrenaline and cortisol hormones that are produced in the brain stimulate the grey matter and improve sharpness of mind.

19

Call Centre Syndrome

This new entity disease is coming in epidemic proportions since the outsourcing of manpower by Multinationals to India. Following are the common entities, patients are suffering from, who had come to me with not only disease as a result of working in the call centres but also associated side-effects of allopathic treatment they had for their symptoms.

A. Cervical Syndrome

The symptoms are typical of cervical spondylosis because of strain on arm and neck muscles. These are pain, numbness, weakness of arm, forearm and finger muscles.

Allopathy

The orthopaedic surgeons give NSAID preparations which cause gastritis, skin allergy and fluid retention.

Homeopathy

I have given them my cocktail of cal.fluor, cimcifuga, ruta, rhus tox and arnica.

In advanced cases, I have given them high potency of causticum.

B. Sleeplessness (Insomnia)

This is due to disturbance in sleep pattern as a result of

shift duties. As a result, there is heaviness of head in the morning.

Allopathy

The allopath physicians often give tranquillizers or sleeping pills which make them addictive and permanent customers of the doctors.

Homeopathy

I give them Passiflora. Inf.-Q 20 to 30 drops, 1 hour before sleep.

C. Gastric Problems

a) Acidity and reflux oesophagitis.
b) Constipation.
c) Indigestion.

These are often due to irregularity in foods and sleep pattern.

Allopathy

They are given zanetac, omez, cremmefin, dulcolax, normaxine and domstal.

I have seen these simply disturb the peristaltic waves rather than establishing equilibrium.

Homeopathy

I often give them asafoetida, iris versicola and carbo veg. for acid reflux.

For constipation, I give them alumina and nux vomica, 200 potency.

For indigestion, I give them antimonaium crudum and hydrastasis.

D. Sexual Debility and Neurosthenia

These develop as a result of inadequate sleep, irritability and depression.

Allopathy

There is nothing to offer.

Homeopathy

I advise them ashwagandha and zincum met and Kali phosphorus.

E. Skin Changes

Due to irregularity in duties and timings, they get dark circles below the eyes due to inadequate sleep and shift duties.

Ashwagandha and vitamins B & C and adequate sleep is the remedy.

F. Headache and Heaviness of Head

Allopathy

Tylenol, combiflam, bruffen are the common medicines but these cause dryness of mouth, gastritis and increase in weight due to fluid retention.

Homeopathy

I often give them Kali phos, Cimcifuga and Onosmodium (due to eye strain) because of working on computers and gelsemium.

G. Noises in Ears and Deafness

Over prolonged periods of working, they get these symptoms and I have seen cases of tumour (acoustic neuroma) behind the ears because of constant use of telephones.

Allopathy

There is nothing to offer.

Homeopathy

I give them Nat.salycylate, Causticum, Chininum Salicylate.

In resistant cases, I give them Kali iodide and Kali muraticum.

20

Vaccinations

There is no doubt that with increase in the number of vaccinations, there is increase in vaccine-related diseases, like autism, chest allergy and skin diseases like eczema.

According to Allopaths, it is considered to be absurd on my part to say that the above diseases are vaccine related.

Homeopaths are strongly against vaccinations at least on paper and in books authored by them.

My personal approach is that vaccinations should be given (only essential ones) and not every year.

My evidence that vaccines cause the above diseases is based on the fact that I have treated these diseases which are vaccine related.

These diseases are coming up in epidemic proportions in western countries and the same in India owing to the fact that more vaccines are given to children.

Recently, even allopaths have admitted that autism in some cases have been traced to mercury used as preservative in some vaccines.

In my experience, influenza vaccine every year is creating more harm than good.

Homeopathic preparations like Thuja, Silicea, Antim tart have never let me down to treat the above conditions.

21

Miscellaneous

ARTERIOSCLEROSIS

A.C.T.

Everybody is aware that incidence of heart disease, high blood pressure and cerebral complications are due to use of excessive fats, that cause hardening and thickening of arteries because of cholesterol and calcareous deposits. This pathological condition is called Arteriosclerosis.

Ideally proper diet and physical exercise go a long way to prevent this condition.

Allopathy

Allopathic drugs, so far available in the world to lower the cholesterol, have highly adverse effects.

Effect of Allopathy

The commonly used anticholesterol drugs (Statins):

1. can affect the liver.
2. can cause muscle degeneration.
3. can cause loss of libido and impotency.
4. can produce chances of gall stone formation.

Keeping this thing in mind, I mention below some of the homeopathic preparations meant to reduce cholesterol and calcarious deposits in the arteries.

Homeopathy

1. Crategus Q, 8 drops in the morning and evening in water after meals for 3-6 months.
2. Cholesterinum 3x 2 pills thrice a day for 3 months.
3. Baryta Carb 200 once a week.
4. Pulsatilla 30 twice daily.
5. Puls 30 and ant.crud 30, if digestion is weak.

ANAEMIA

A.C.T.

It is a very common condition, more so in Asian and African countries due to poor diet.

1. Find out and treat the cause.
2. In most cases, the cause is not known, especially in cases of women and children.

Allopathy

The frequent side-effects of these iron preparations are as follows:

1. Diarrhoea, constipation, gastric pain.
2. Headache or allergic skin reaction.
3. There are cases where iron preparations are not assimilated.
4. These may be absorbed and may cause liver problem by depositing there.

Homeopathy

Ferrum Phos 6x and Lecithine ½ to 2 grains or 30 potency, preferably in crude form.

BLEEDING (Haemorrhage)

This chapter excludes the bleeding from Gynae causes which has been dealt with at length later on.

Bleeding from any orifice or any organ. Allopathic haemostatic agents can cause disastrous side-effects on blood pressure and heart, especially if the patient's condition is very critical or elderly patients have poor cardiac function. In such circumstances, homeopathy is safe and patient-friendly. Replacement of fluids is a must, wherever necessary.

My experience with allopathic and homeopathic haemostatic agents in each type of bleeding is illustrated in the following cases:

Nose Bleeding

Allopathy

I have used Revici or Dicynene for 20 years but I had many cases where it failed to stop the bleeding (excluding big vessel or hypertension as the cause).

In India, I have used Botropase and Styptobion and both are quite effective, but disseminated intravascular clotting as a complication with Botropase should not be ignored. Andrenochrome, years ago, was very popular in U.K. but had deleterious effects on heart and blood pressure.

Homeopathy

Locally: Calendula Q + Trillium Q is very very useful. *Internally:* Arnica, Bryonia and Aconite are often very helpful. I have tried this cocktail in hundreds of cases and it has never let me down.

Eye Intraoccular or Retinal Bleeding

This condition is becoming increasingly common these days, due to diabetes, hypertension and on being on aspirin for a long-term as a cardiac or stroke prevention.

Allopathy

As often the case, I find Aspirin, when taken for a long-time (as with other drugs), it overshoots the mark. I have seen hundreds of cases with epistaxis in ear, nose and throat department, due to aspirin. The same way there has been bleeding in middle ear due to aspirin. Patients come with sudden deafness and no pain. They complain of blocked feeling. The G.P. had already syringed their ears considering the dark membrane as wax.

In general practice, I have seen lot of cases of haematuria (bleeding in urine) or Haematemesis (bleeding from gastrointestinal tract). For the same reason, bleeding in retina due to aspirin also causes blurring of vision.

In retinal bleeding, no doubt, laser gives immediately gratifying results but only for short periods. Moreover, not many centres are equipped with this expertise or equipment in India. These patients are often on anti-inflammatory drugs for arthritis and these drugs also contribute to bleeding. One should try to find the cause by history or investigations and blood tests. Sometimes the cause is generalised disease.

Case I

I remember years ago as a casualty officer in England, I confronted a young girl of 22 years coming with severe vaginal bleeding. After I put the vaginal pack which stopped the vaginal bleeding, she had nasal bleeding. As I had done E.N.T. house job prior to casualty, I used my expertise to pack the nose.

In retrospect, had I known homeopathy at that time, I would have treated such a case with homeopathy which would have worked at both ends.

Homeopathy

Following homeopathic remedies have been of unquestionable value in many such types of cases. The remedies which I have used extensively recently, where nasal packing and cautery have failed, are as given below:

1. Hammamelis
2. Millifolium
3. Trillium
4. Phosphorus

5. Calendula 30
6. Fucus religiosa
7. Blumia
8. Arnica

These drugs have given me gratifying results. These I have given internally. At the same time, I have used mother tinctures of these locally.

In E.N.T. operations where allopathic haemostatic drugs have failed or their side-effects outweigh the risks, these homeopathic preparations I have used locally with immense benefit.

In secondary bleeding, which occurs 5-7 days after operation or after any injury incurred a few days prior to bleeding, such bleeding, especially with pyrexia, is due to bacterial infection. Here I have given antibiotics internally; while locally I have used Calendula-Q and Crotalus Horridus 6x diluted in distilled water. I have found at times severe reaction in sensitive persons to betadine.

Allopathy

Often these have systemic side-effects.

Homeopathy

Crotalus Horridus 6x potency is very effective. The characteristic indication of this remedy is dark blood. Sometimes in septic haemorrhagic condition, it is the ideal.

CHICKEN POX

Being a common infectious disease, often no treatment is given, but when the symptoms of itching are very severe with threatened superadded infection, it needs medications.

Allopathy

This does interfere with the normal course of disease. Antibiotics at times had to be given if there is superadded infection. In such circumstances, there is a possibility of allergic reaction to the antibiotics. Antiallergic drugs are given to control itching.

Homeopathy

In contrast, homeopathy controls all the symptoms. Rhus tox 30, 3-4 hourly is excellent to control the itching and, at the same time, prevents infection of the vesicles of chicken pox. If itching is associated with cough and vomiting, then Antim tart 4 times a day is given.

COLD SORE (Herpes Simplex)

It is a very common condition, especially occurring in people with low resistance.

Allopathy

Anti-allergic or anti-inflammatory preparations simply cause drowsiness and stomatitis.

Homeopathy

Rhus tox 30 alternating with Dulcamara 30 often controls this condition.

HERPES ZOSTER

A.C.T.

It may involve any nerve, but common ones are nasociliary, trigemial, and intercostal.

Allopathy

Zovirax is specific for this condition both locally and systemically, but therapeutic doses cannot be tolerated by everybody.

Effect of Allopathy

After the acute stage is over, the neuralgia and, at times

numbness, is most annoying. Strong allopathic pain-killer is hardly a cure for post-herpetic neuralgia.

Homeopathy

Apis 30, Rhus tox 30, Belladona 30 in cyclic rotation. In post-therapeutic and neuralgia, Mezerium 30, 3-4 hourly.

HEEL PAIN

It is one of the commonest and annoying conditions. It is at the attachment of Tendo Archillis at Calcaneum bone.

Allopathy

X-ray often shows the shadow of the spur. Orthopaedic surgeons often give injection at the local site.

Effect of Allopathy

Apart from side-effects of steroids, it is only a temporary relief-giving measure.

Homeopathy

Arnica 200, Cimcifuga 30, Ruta 30 in cyclic rotation. Sometimes Thuja 200, 1M as intercurrent medicine.

DEBILITY

Homeopathic treatment for debility is tailor-made unlike pushing the vitamins and preparations in allopathic way of treating.

Homeopathy

1. Due to Anaemia : Already mentioned.
2. After any acute illness like influenza, typhoid : Lyco 30, carbo veg 200, 1M
3. After Allopathic medicines : Nit.acid, nux.vom 30
4. After any drainage China 30 + Carbo Veg 30

illness like diarrhoea, seminal emissions, leucorrhoea	: Acid phos 30 alternating with veratrum alb. 200 vomiting and loss of blood
5. After mental strain leading to physical weakness	: Acid phos 30,200
6. After sexual intercourse	: Acid phos 30, china 30, selenium 30 in cyclic rotation.

INSOMNIA (Sleeplessness)

It is becoming an ailment in epidemic form owing to modern stresses and strains and less physical activity.

Allopathy

Calmpose, Larpose, Ativan, Alzolam, Librax, Hynotex and hoard of other sedatives.

Effect of Allopathy

Long-term use of these sedatives has the following disadvantages beyond doubt:

1. **Habit forming** whatever the manufacturers may mention on the contrary.
2. **Depression** with Calmpose and Valium. After a few years, these patients had to go on to anti-depressants.
3. **Parkinsonism** is again the commonest disease afflicting people especially on tranquillisers and antihypertensive drugs.
4. **Hepatotoxicity** in prolonged use of allopathic medicines.

The homeopathy is tailor-made in cases of insomnia.

The following table gives the list of homeopathic medicines depending upon the causes:

Cause of Insomnia	Remedy
1. No apparent cause	Alfa Q + Crategus Q +

	Passiflora Q (1 : 1 : 3) 10 to 15 drops tds. in water.
2. Due to anxiety, grief and worries	Coffea 30 + Gel 30 + Kali phos 30, 2 doses, 2 hourly before going to bed.
3. Due to some pain	Opium 30, 200.

OBESITY

A.C.T.

It is a fatty condition due to accumulation of excessive fat. It is caused by the following factors:

1. By consumption of more food than required to produce energy.
2. Sometimes, women develop obesity due to frequent abortions and operations; even minor, due to transfusion of normal or saline blood.
3. Some allopathic drugs without the patient realising the cause, like NSAID preparations. These cause obesity by causing retention of fluids in the body.
4. Anti-tubercular drugs by causing changes in fat metabolism.
5. Steroids and Sibellium (for migrain) are top culprits for causing obesity.
6. Hormonal imbalance is another cause, Myxoedema (Thyroid deficiency), Oestrogen preparations for irregular periods.
7. Contraceptive pills often lead to obesity.

Allopathy

Various preparations like Ponderax are very favourite with women.

Effect of Allopathy

1. Depression and dependance are the most worst side-effects of Ponderax (Fenfluramine).

2. Gastrointestinal disturbances (Flatulence, constipation)
3. Irritability, hypotension, urinary frequency.
4. Impotency, loss of libido.
5. Schizophrenic like reactions (Delusions, Hallucinations and sleep disturbances) are common.

Homeopathy

For different types of obesity:

1. Obesity in women with weak heart, dyspnoea, wheezing.	Calcarea arsenic 30, Apis 30.
2. General obesity, large abdomen, sesitive to cold.	Calc.carb. 30, twice daily.
3. Post-operative (D&C, caesarean etc.)	Thyroid 6x and apis 30, each twice daily.
4. Obesity with joint pains. (vicious cycle)	Calc.carb 30, alt.colch. 30, twice each.

The key to secret of reducing weight is that input should be less than output and yogic exercises.

HEALTH & SEX (MISCELLANEOUS)

My three basic principles for good health which I advise to my patients are:
1. Good sleep.
2. Good nutritional, balanced food.
3. Active sexual life taking in healthy spirit of necessity rather than a liability.

Since the publishing of my last edition, new research and new developments in the field of sex and health have taken place. In that context, I would also like to mention the result of homeopathic remedies in sexual health, both in men and women.

It will not be out of place to bring to the notice of the readers, the views of experts in the field of sexual health.

Michael Roizen views published in BMJ titled "**SEX AND DEATH: Are They Related**":

The more the orgasm and the more often the sex, the healthier is the effect on health. This is in contrast to the word often used by Homeopaths in their books, that sex is synonymous to sins. Even they usually label masturbation as a sin and they usually advise Staph. for such acts. Being an allopath and homeopath, I strongly condemn the word **sins** used by homeopaths in their books.

In my practice, I have seen many patients especially who are religious, more so in Asian countries, sex is a taboo and such patients have poor health in contrast to those who take it as a necessity. I agree with Cynthia Watson M.D. and author of "A guide to Aphrodisiacs and Sexual Pleasures". Healthy sexual life and health are intrinsingly related. Sex makes you relax, relieves stress, and produces endorphins. Sex helps the immune system better.

Allopathy & A.C.T.

Those who suffer from impotency, which is becoming very common even in young people, Viagra and Levitra are good preparations but these do not increase the desire or the libido, these simply cause erection.

The common cause for impotency in young people is either psychological or who are diabetic or on antihypertensive drugs.

The adverse effects of viagra should not be underestimated. These especially lead to low blood pressure and can be dangerous in patients who are on coronary vasodilators and antihypertensive drugs.

Tidalafil and Levitra are better than viagra. The onset of action is smooth, duration of action is 36 hours with Tidalafil and Levitra.

Homeopathy

In young people, Psychotherapy, Lycopodium (not to be repeated frequently), Damiana-Q and Yohimbine (piles must be excluded) are often successful.

Allopathy & Homeopathy

In certain patients who really bent upon taking Levitra, I counteract the hypotensive effect of Levitra by giving Viscum-Q, Carbo. veg and China.

It is true that Levitra is really a weekend pill since the action lasts for 36 to 48 hours. The onset of action is smooth. The side-effects due to vasodilatation are far less severe than encountered with Viagra. Levitra, which goes by the name of Cialis in UK and USA, is the most popular Recently, I have seen the combination of Ashwagandha, Muira-puama and Yohimbine acts as a "sex bomb" with increase in desire also. The patients told me that Viagra was no comparison to these. But one big disadvantage with Muria-puama, Yohimbine, Damiana is that these cause haemorrhoids (piles) which Tidalafil does not.

IMPOTENCY

A.C.T.

There is no full erection of penis to enter vagina or when there is quick ejaculation of semen as soon as penis enters vagina.

Common **causes** are: 1. Diabetes; 2. Anti-hypertensive Drugs; 3. Masturbation; 4. Excessive coitus; or 5. Psychological problems like depression and fear.

Allopathy

It should not be used, especially Testosterone preparations. **Complications and adverse effects due to hormones** taken for impotency:

1. Renal, 2. Cardiac, 3. Hepatic complications, 4. Hypercalcaemia leading to kidney stones, 5. Prostatic cancer is another complication which can occur, 6. Sodium retention, oedema and increase in weight, breast cancer in men.

VIAGRA (Sildenafil)

No doubt, this preparation by Pfizer has revolutionised the progress. But one must keep in mind the following dark signals when taking this preparation.

a. Often men who need this preparation are diabetic or hypertensive and are taking CORONARY dilators which also lower the blood pressure and can initiate Heart stroke.
b. Secondly, Viagra does not increase desire. It only causes erection.

In contrast, in Homeopathy, Yohimbine, Nuphar Agnus & Acid Phos increase the desire and erection in a natural way.

Homeopathy

1. Lycopodium 1M, 10M, once a month. No other medicines that day and a day after. Lycopodium is useful especially for elderly men.
2. Staphysagaria 30, 200, for men who develop impotency as a result of masturbation.
3. Acid Phos 30, 200 for most of the cases belonging to this category, where fear and apprehension is the cause of being unable to rise to the occasion.
4. China 30, 200 as a result of debilitating illness with loss of fluids.
5. Selenium 30, 200 as a result of onanism and secret vice.
6. Idiopathic Impotency: Tribules-Terr Q (8-10 drops in water) after meals, 2-3 times a day and Yohimbine Q (8-10 drops in water) after meals.

But Yohimbine should not be given in cases of gastritis and haemorrhoids, since both these conditions can flare up with Yohimbine.

SEX, BRAIN AND HOMEOPATHY

As a German researcher, Werner Habermehl has said, sex stimulates the brain and makes people more intelligent. Habermehl, who works at Hamburg Research Institute, claims that regular sexual intercourse promotes intelligence. He says love-making, besides physically exciting the body, also provides brain with plenty of excitement. This consequently increases the amount of adrenaline and cortisol hormones that are produced in the brain, stimulates the grey matter and improves the sharpness of mind.

Homeopathy

My experience with homeopathic Aphrodisiac remedies on patients have certainly increased their happiness in sexual life and definitely sharpness of mind, compared to those on allopathy. The commonly given remedies are Agnus, Lycopodium and Caladium and Muira-puama.

SCIATICA

A.C.T.

This is becoming a very common ailment owing to sedentary life, lack of exercise and bad posture, sometimes due to injection at the wrong site.

Allopathy

During **acute** stage: Analgesics, physiotherapy, diathermy, traction, bed rest.

But since analgesics are to be used for longer period and also for relapses, again and again, adverse and toxic effects are very very bad (see under diseases caused by allopathic treatment).

Homeopathy

In most cases, where I have been called to see them, are those who had undergone surgery for prolapsed disc or analgesics have caused mouth ulcers, gastritis and haemorrhoids. During **acute** condition:

1. Acute stage	: Cimcifuga, colocynth, belladona, mag phos 30 in cyclic rotation never lets me down.
2. In cases of associated nerve symptoms of numbness, paraesthesia	: Gnaphallium, bryonia often helps.
3. Sciatica with low BP	: Crategus Q + Cactus Q.
4. Sciatica worst at rest, in cold weather, rainy season and coughing	: Rhus tox 200.

MILK SUPPRESSION IN LACTATING WOMEN

1. Due to emotional disturbances: Cimcifuga 30,200.
2. Non-appearance without any apparent cause: Causticum, Ricinus, Communis Lecithine 3x or 4x 3 times daily.
3. Swollen and painful breasts but no milk: Pulsatilla 30.

LACTATION AFTER WEANING

This is the most challenging to Gynae.-Obs. surgeons. The only remedy with them is Hormone Treatment which has tremendous side-effects. Even the tests alone for hormones are beyond the reach of middle class.

Homeopathy

Lac can 30,200 has been successful in 90% of the cases. So far, I have treated ten such cases ranging between ages of 24 and 32 years.

FATIGUE

A.C.T.

Allopathy

Often in allopathy we give vitamins or tranquillisers and advise physical rest.
Practically, these three modes of treatment are not tenable.

Effect of Allopathy

1. Tranquillisers affect alertness.
2. Time is too precious these days and one cannot take off work since that will affect earnings.
3. Vitamins will not always help. Proper diet is better than the intake of vitamins. Some are allergic to vitamins.

Homeopathy

It is tailor-made for fatigue:

1. If physically tired	:	Arnica 200.
2. If mentally tired like students and thinkers	:	Anacardium 30,200, Kaliphos 6x.
3. General bodily fatigue	:	Ginsen Q.
4. On least exertion	:	Picric Acid.
5. Mental & physical exertion	:	Arg. Nit, Acid phos.
6. Due to any other cause	:	Sterculia.

EPILEPSY

Tegratol (Carbamazepine) is a common life-saving drug used in epilepsy and trigeminal neuralgia. Often its use had to be advised for a long time owing to nature of illness. A few cases on tegratol with the following complications:
Homeopathic treatment for tegratol complications:

a. Ulcerative colitis	: Merc sol colocynth, Mag phos, Cup met phos, Cup met.
b. Nephritis	: Berberis Q and Sarsaprilla.

c. Psychosis : Aurum met, Kali phos.
d. Arrythmias : Crategus Q + Cactus Q and Abies n.

COMPLEXION

A.C.T.

It should not be misunderstood that homeopathy can change the complexion in every case. But the following case that came to me is worth mentioning.

Case

A lady, aged 42 years, came to me with a complaint that after taking Sparfloxacine from a doctor for trivial complaint of acute bronchitis, she developed dark complexion due to photosensitive and loss of smell. These side-effects of quinolone, though not common, are not rare either. Another patient came with loss of smell after spar.

Allopathically, there is no treatment for both these side-effects.

Homeopathy

Iodium 1000, one dose a fortnight brought her complexion back and Anacardium 200 for loss of smell.

FACIAL HAIR IN WOMEN (Hirsuitism)

This condition is becoming increasingly common unlike three decades ago. Probably, it is a nature's competition with opening of increasing number of cosmetic and beauty parlours.

Often it is labelled as hereditary, but that is not true since I could not find any clinical evidence on that ground.

However, there is definite link of hirsuitism due to increasing number of hormonal preparations given for various menstrual problems, though those menstrual problems could be due to stress and strain.

Another common cause for this condition is every other physician or gynae-obs. gives one or the other form of steroids which lead to hirsuitism.

Again at menopause, I find lot of women develop hirsuitism due to hormonal changes.

Allopathy

The common line of treatments undertaken by girls are at beauty parlours by electrolysis which do lead, at times, to scarring and also certain marks and still I have not found it giving permanent results.

The other line of treatment by cosmetic surgeons, which, apart from certain limitations in good results, are not within the reach of everybody, being expensive.

Homeopathy

I commence my treatment with Thuja 1M. I have seen somehow that 200 potency does not work in this ailment. Then after gving a gap of 2 days, I give oleum jec 3x or 30 depending upon the weather.

Every homeopath is familiar with this regime, but I find Sepia and Ovarian extract preparation 3x by Bhandari Chemists, over a period of time gives good results.

Case I

Miss B, 22 years old, a computer post-graduate student, came to me with the following symptoms:

1. Amenorrhoea, 4 years since entry into professional college.
2. Facial hair for last 3 years, since she had been on hormonal treatment for amenorrhoea.
3. Tremendous increase in weight for the last 3 years.
4. High blood pressure for the last 2 years.
5. Depression for the last 1 year.

Now here is a girl who has been victim of the so to say modern treatment by hormones for amenorrhoea by top gynaecologists.

Allopathy

There is nothing what could have been done. The most depressing thing was that amenorrhoea was still persistent after she stopped hormonal treatment owing to their side-effects.

Homeopathy Reasons

1. Firstly, I treated her depression with Ignatia and Aurum met.
2. Then I treated her fluid retention and consequent increase in weight with Stropanthus and Apis.
3. Then I treated her high blood pressure with Raulwofia+Crategus and Passiflora.
4. Finally, I treated her amenorrhoea and facial hair, commencing with Thuja and going to Pulsatilla and Sepia.

   It took six months before this lady was brought to 80% normal in all her symptoms when I had to go abroad for assignment.

PERSPIRATION

Normal perspiration should not be arrested but when the perspiration is pathological as given under, then the treatment should be as follows:

Allopathy

All the anti-perspirants available are dangerous and may cause suppression hazards, apart from local allergic reactions.

Homeopathy

1. If excessive, then Kali Carb 30, 4 hourly.
2. If offensive, then Nitric Acid 30, 4 hourly.
3. If it is garlic odour perspiration, then Lycopodium.

ACUTE LUMBAGO WITH SCIATICA

A cousin of mine, 55 years old, suffered from severe lower backache with sciatica on left side. In addition to the backache, she had acute osteoarthritis of left knee joint. She was extremely restless, unable to take a turn in bed, feeling very weak.

Investigations: X-ray lumbosacral and knee joint revealed slight reduction of lumbosacral space, some degree of osteoporosis, no abnormality of knee joint, blood tests excluded, multiple myeloma or any tubercular or secondaries.

Allopathy

Heavy doses of Diclofen, Proxyvon had only slight benefit, which was of short duration. Severe gastritis ocurred despite giving antacid preparations like ranitidine. Even two weeks of allopathic treatment did not make noticeable difference.

Homeopathy

It is tailor-made and very specific. For backache and sciatica: Kali Carb 30 alternate with Cimcifuga 30 had a magical effect. Then I increased to Cimcifuga 200 and one dose a day, Kali Carb 200 one dose a day had cured the backache almost 95% in 48 hours. For left knee joint osteoarthritis, I gave Ruta 30 alternate with Argentum metallicum 30 and Bryonia 30 in cyclic rotation.

To finish the cure, I gave Colchicum 200 (AM), Ruta 200 (noon), Rhus tox 200 (evening), Argentum metallicum 200 at night. Physiotherapy for knee muscles and spine muscles was advised to prevent relapses.

BED SORES

All specialists have encountered this condition at one time or the other.

Allopathy

Locally antiseptic, antibiotic powders are, no doubt, of great help but, in my experience, I have found the use of homeopathy as complementary to allopathy.

Locally: Calendula Q and Hypericum Q.

Internally: Calendula and Hypericum should be taken in 30 potency.

PROLAPSE UTERUS, DEPRESSION, HALLUCINATIONS, DELUSIONS AND REFLUX OESOPHAGITIS

Mrs. K, an 80-year-old lady, was brought to me which, in my life time, I had seen the worst type of uterus prolapse. The prolape was of the size of a medium-sized apple. She had been treated at two top hospitals of Delhi, but the gynae-obs. tried pessaries which will not retain there, she was unfit for operation.

I was not keen to take over this case since prognosis seemed to be poor, but on insistence of her devoted daughter-in-law, I accepted.

She also had been on antidepressant and sleeping pills which made her confused with loss of orientation of space and time apart from gastric problems.

A.C.T.

Homeopathy

1. For uterus prolapse, I gave her Sepia, Podophyllum and acid nitric in increasing potency every week.
2. After 4 weeks, I put her on Calc. fl and Aloe for the prolapse.
3. For her hallucinations and delusions, I put her on Hyoscamus and Strammonium.
4. For her memory and confusion, I put her on Baryta carb and Ambra in increasing potencies.

It took me 3 months, and now she is not on any allopathic medicines and she is 50% better in all aspects and easy to be managed by her daughter-in law.

ATTENTION DEFICIENT DISORDER & ATTENTION DEFICIENT HYPERACTIVE DISORDER

These two conditions are becoming very common all over the world today.

Challenging problems are being faced by the parents of such children, teachers, psychologists and paediatricians.

I will deal with these two conditions under different headings.

Attention Deficient Disorder

The child exhibits delays in reading, maths skills, spelling, writing or difficulty with comprehension and retention of material (Dyslexia) or becomes a slow learner.

Very often the children have been brought to me after the parents noticed side-effects of allopathic drug RITALIN given for attention deficient disorder. Psychologists and paediatricians and teachers have tried their best but failed.

A.C.T.

The beneficial results with homeopathy are noticed as follow:

1. The teachers will notice a distinct change in your child's learning skills.
2. The child will report more ease and less frustration with learning. He/she will no longer feel school-going and doing homework as a struggle.
3. School grades improve significantly.
4. Behaviour will improve remarkably.
5. Handwriting will become more legible.
6. Finally, the child will spontaneously enjoy reading which he/she previously used to feel as a burden.

I have noticed these changes occur within three to six weeks. To me it has given me extreme pleasure to hear in the words of the child, telling me how much easier school has become and how they love being a part of it. The treatment should be under an experienced homeopath.

1. **Baryta Carb** is the head remedy. Most of the milestones are slow and delayed in such cases. There is varying degree of backwardness in such cases.

2. **Calcarea Carb:** I have treated many cases successfully with it. Head sweating, chubby and fair complexion children respond very well to Calcarea Carb as exemplified in the following case.

Case I

A seven-year-old girl, with a history of Attention Deficient Disorder, skin allergies and bed wetting, came to me.

She was fair complexion, chubby girl and good in memorising but easily got distracted and she was also an egg and cheese lover. In the first week, I gave her Calcarea Carb 30 twice a day and Calcarea Carb 200 once a week.

She became a totally different child in six weeks' time.

Attention Deficient Hyperactive Disorder

Case II

This is a very interesting case of a sixteen-year-old boy, whose parents got him treated in U.S.A. and Germany for his following symptons:

1. Fair complexion, disobedient, arrogant, rude and disinterested in studies.
2. Easily distracted.
3. More interested in friends than in studies.
4. He is intelligent but channelising his energy not in studies but music and other activities. He has hyperflexible joints and used to get vomiting and stomachache feeling whenever he used to go to school in early childhood.

5. He had many destructive habits such as burning paper, cutting papers into small pieces and nail biting.
6. At times, he had stealing habits, for which he had been reprimanded in school.

Allopathy

He was given RITALIN after which the child started developing side-effects like high blood pressure and on withdrawal of RITALIN, the child went into depression. At this stage, the parents sought my advice for giving homeopathy.

Homeopathy

I gave Calcarea Phos. first week, 30 potency twice a day, next week 200 for alternate days. This was given because of excessive flexibility of joints and certain prominence of chest bones.

In the second week, I gave Veratrum Alb. 200 on alternate days in the morning. **This was given for the symptoms of cutting paper.**

Every night Kali Phos. 30 was given to soothen the nerves.

Conclusion:

The positive response with these remedies were observed in the following criteria:

(a) Got interested in studies and started enjoying doing it.
(b) Less distraction.
(c) Improved in grades.
(d) Became more responsible.

22

Cautions in Homeopathy

1. Lay persons, who profess Homeopaths, should be careful in using **high** potencies which can act as a **double-edged knife**.

2. **Examination** of the patient is important. It is completely ridiculous to make a diagnosis on the basis of symptoms alone. Recently, I had seen a patient with pain in the mastoid region being treated by eminent homeopaths, one after the other, putting the patient on Capsicum and Phosphorus for six months. The patient came to my clinic with symptoms of prolonged use of Capsicum. There was clinically absolutely no sign of mastrioditis at all. It was a pain due to C. spondylosis.

3. Any **surgical** cause of disease, such as big perforation in ear, deviated nasal bone, should be treated surgically. So, a specialist examination, if needed, must be carried out before treating homeopathically.

4. **Investigations**, where necessary, must be carried out before arriving at any conclusion.

5. I have seen most homeopaths laying stress on symptoms alone for treating their patients. With the availability of advanced diagnostic tools, proper diagnosis must be decided by thorough examination. If we go only on symptoms, does it mean that many symptom-free diseases

like hypertension, tumours of breast should need no treatment according to homeopathic approach to disease?

6. **It is a misconception in the mind of a layman – and even in the mind of some homeopaths – that homeopathy is absolutely safe. Incorrect potency, its prolonged and wrong treatment can definitely lead to innumerable diseases.**

A few examples given below will suffice to make the people cautious:

a. A patient came to me with acute left frontal and maxillary sinusitis, saying that she was given 10M Silicea for her rheumatic pain. X-ray showed left maxillary and left frontal sinusitis. She had excruciating pain on left side of the head around the left eyeball with danger of meningitis. I did the emergency drainage of the sinusitis. There was another danger of giving high potency of Silicea to such a patient since she had treated T.B. of lungs which can flare up with Silicea.

b. I have seen hoards of examples of giving Hepar Sulph or taking on their own for tonsillitis. I have seen cases of provings and high potency given frequently, leading to abscess of tonsils. There are many tonsil preparations available in the market which are considered to be harmless but that is not the case. Hepar Sulph should also be given with caution in the case of old T.B.

c. Tuberculinum is the remedy used very often by professionals and laymen indiscriminately. I have seen many cases developing T.B. abcess because of its indiscriminate use.

d. **Thuja** is a wonderful drug if used after knowing the proper symptoms. I have seen a patient being given either a high or low potency for a nasal polyp by a highly reputed homeopath without seeing the nose resulting in various side-effects.

CAUTIONS

It is a misconception in people's mind that homeopathy is absolutely safe. Of course, compared to other branches of medicine like allopathy and ayurveda, homeopathy is safer.

But when used by amateur people without experience, many problems come up. I have seen the following types of cases created by homeopathy:

Prolonged Use

Too long use of the remedy leads to proving effect. Many inexperienced homeopaths or patients themselves keep on taking the medicine with the hope that beneficial effect will come after some time.

High Potency

This should be used by an experienced homeopath. High potency can act as a double-edged knife, if not used cautiously. It can aggravate the condition to an irreversible stage.

I do not mean that one should not use high potency. To get a cure in certain diseases one has to use high potency, but it must be used by an experienced homeopath.

Wrong Remedy

Certain remedies are contra-indicated in certain conditions. Not only symptoms but full diagnosis should be made and thorough physical examination should be done, for example:

1. Hepar Sulph should be used with caution in old cases of T.B.
2. Silicea should not be used in an old case of T.B.
3. Phosphorus should be used with caution in T.B.

I know a case of a 50-year-old lady, who was given very high potency of Silicea to treat a case of simple tonsillitis by a top homeopath professor with the hope that it will burst. The patient came with acute respiratory distress to me after the quinsy has ruptured into lateral pharyngeal space.

It was really a problem to get the name of remedy that the professor had given. I gave the patient following treatment:

1. Antidote to Silicea
2. Drainage of lateral pharyngeal abscess.
3. Calendula 30, 4 times a day, internally.

Sulphur is being used very indiscriminately. Various severe reactions have occurred when used by inexperienced homeopaths.

Aconite

1. Do not use in malarial fever, pyrexic conditions, fever with eruptions.
2. Do not use if its mental symptoms, i.e., anxiousness, restlessness of mind and body are not present.

Aloe Socot

Do not repeat frequently in rectal conditions. Wait after a few doses.

Alumina

Do not change early as the action of this drug is slow in developing.

Ammonium Carb

1. Do not use in low potency.
2. Do not use before or after lachesis.

Anacardium

Do not use where there is excessive coagulability of blood.

Antim Tart

1. Do not forget that when Thuja fails, Silicea is contraindicated on bad effects of vaccination.
2. Do not forget Hepar Sulph when Antim Tart seems indicated but fails.

Apis Mel

1. Do not use in low potency, too frequently or for long in pregnancy, especially around 3rd month. It may cause abortion if given around that time.
2. Do not change hastily, as sometimes its action is slow, especially when diuretic action is sought for.
3. Do not use before or after Rhus tox.

Arnica Mont

1. Do not apply at all when abraision or cuts are present. It may produce severe erysipelas for which condition Camphor comes to our rescue.
2. Do not use externally or internally in case of a mad dog bite.

Baryta Carb

1. Do not use in Catarrhal Asthma.
2. Do not give low potency. Use in highest potencies to remove the predisposition to quinsy.

Belladona

1. Do not use in acute appendicitis, even if symptoms are free.
2. Do not use in higher potencies, it may kill the patient.
3. Do not use in Typhoid or continuous fever.

Bellis Per

Do not give at bed time. It causes Insomnia.

Benzoic Acid

Do not take alcohol after it. It will aggravate Genty, Rheumatic and Urinary infections.

Blatta Oṛi

Do not repeat after the attack, if improvement continues. It may bring unnecessary aggravation in such cases.

Bryonia

Remember that it has Alumina for its chronic stage.

Caladium

Do not forget that it destroys craving for tobacco.

Calcarea Carb

1. Do not use before Baryta Carb or Kali Bio.
2. Do not use after Kali Carb.
3. Do not forget that it is chronic of Belladona.

Camphor

1. Do not allow in the sick room in crude form as it antidotes most of the vegetable medicines.
2. Do not use in water as it aggravates.
3. Do not use if there is sweat or stop it as soon as sweat occurs.

Carbo Veg

Do not use in early stage of any disease whatsoever, especially in Diarrhoea.

Causticum

Do not use too frequently in paralytic infections; only once or twice a week.

Chamomilla

Do not use if the patient is calm and quiet.

China

1. Do not use below 200 in nervous and irritable children.
2. Do not forget that Santo may cure worms if China fails.
3. Do not forget that it has cured Aphonia from exposure if Aco, Phos has failed.

Colchicum

Do not forget that it cures Oedema when Apis fails.

Collinsonia

1. Do not use low where there is an organic heart disease.
2. Do not forget in Colic when Colocynth and Nux have failed.

Crategus

Do not change in haste. Should be used for some time to obtain good results.

Hepar Sulph

Do not use in Coryza in the beginning if it is likely to drive the trouble to chest.

Ignatia

1. Do not use at bed time. It may cause Insomnia.

Kali Bio

1. Do not use after Calcarea Carb.

Kali Carb

1. Do not repeat too often.

2. Do not start with high in old Gout, T.B. or advanced Bright's disease.

Lachesis

1. Do not repeat frequently.
2. Do not use in high potencies without caution.

Lycopodium

Do not use after Sulphur.

Medorrhanum

1. Do not use lower than 200 potency. Higher potencies are to be preferred.
2. Do not repeat often.

Mercurius

Do not use early in tonsillitis.

Nat Mur

Do not use during attack of headache, even if indicated. Paliate the headache first with its acute, namely Bryonia and Nux Vom. Later on, give Natrum Mur for curative effects.

Nitric Acid

1. Do not change or substitute if skin symptoms appear during treatment of some chronic disease. It is a favourable indication.
2. Do not forget that it relieves ailments resulting from abuse of Merc.

Nux Vom

1. Do not give in the morning as it will aggravate the condition.

2. Do not forget to use it when all medicines disagree. It will often cure morbid sensitiveness and other inexplicable troubles.

Passiflora

1. Do not be a miser, give large doses of mother tincture.
2. Do not use high potency in T.B. It may cause haemophysis.

Pulsatilla

1. Do not forget silicea as it is chronic.
2. Do not forget for anaemic and chlorotic patients. It is best against overdosing with iron and tonics, even years before, also at ailments due to excessive tea drinking.

Rhus Tox

1. Do not give before or after Apis.
2. Do not give it to a hot patient even if it exactly corresponds to the symptoms.

Selenium

1. Use neither too low nor repeat too frequently.
2. Do not give in the morning.

Silicea

1. Do not give too low or too high in T.B.
2. Do not use before or after Merc.

Sulphur

1. Do not use in acute abdominal pain.
2. Do not repeat too often.
3. Do not use before Lycopodium.
4. Do not forget it is chronic of Aconite.

Thuja

Do not repeat often. One dose or occasional dose is all that is required.

Thyroidinium

Do not use in tubercular patients.

Tuberculinum

1. Do not use below 200.
2. Do not give without careful examination of heart and lungs.

Veratrum Alb

Do not give below 6th potency in diarrhoea.

FREQUENTLY ASKED QUESTIONS

The common perception held by doctors who had voiced their reservation in homeopathy is that they had the medicines tested (in most cases, given to them by reputed doctors) and it was found to be positive for **cortisone (steroid)**.
1. If one has been on long-term cortisone, one would show cushing syndrome (moon face, excessive body hair, osteoporosis and diabetes).
2. Using steroids in homeopathy will, in fact, be counter-productive as they have suppressing effect. So, considering the above facts, why would any homeopath want to use cortisone? To remove these misconceptions and these allegations, I had discussed with the Biochemists over here and abroad as regards the detailed procedure of testing for steroids. Lactose (milk sugar) is a base for most of the homeopathic medicines. Lactose gives positive test for steroid. So obviously, homeopathic medicines in lactose pills will give a false positive test for steroids. The test used was the colorimetric method using tetrazolium blue salts. In this test, their action depends upon the reduction of tetrazolium blue salt to give a highly coloured compound

known as Farmazan. The amount of Farmazan developed is proportional to the quantity of steroid or any reducing sugar present in the material being tested. So, if the drug contains any lactose, it will impart a strong colour with tetrazolium blue salt which will give a false impression of the presence of a steroid. Secondly, if the alcohol used in this method is not completely free from aldehyde, it will interfere with the reaction and impart some characteristic colour, which may again give false positive reaction for steroid. So, this method is not advisable to determine the presence of steroids in the drug. Most homeopaths use lactose as a base for holding the pills containing the homeopathic remedy. Almost all homeopathic remedies have alcohol as a diluting agent. One can see how homeopathic remedies, either as pills, powders or in alcohol are likely to give false positive test for steroids, if this method is used.

Other methods used to test steroids are Liberman Buchard test (thin layer chromatography method and UV absorption method). Almost all steroids show UV absorption between 235 NM and 240 NM in dehydrated alcohol.

A complete spectrum of this solution is taken between 400 NM and 220 NM. If any steroid is present then it will show maximum at 240 NM. The homeopathic medicines were tested on UV absorption and none of the samples showed maximum between 230 NM and 250 NM indicating absence of steroids.

The same samples, when adulterated with a steroid, showed maximum at 235 NM. Thus, it is clear that before accepting a claim that the tested medicine does contain a steroid, one must find out what testing procedures were used to eliminate the possibility of misleading result.

Q. Any side-effects of homeopathy?

Ans. Yes, if used for too long periods or taken in very high potency.

Q. Can it go with Allopathy?

Ans. Some remedies can go while others are antidotal and complementary.

Q. Can the patient take onion or garlic while taking homeopathic medicines?

Ans. It depends on the type of remedy. Some can be taken while others like all. cepa, onion should be avoided.

Q. How long can it retain its potency?

Ans. Usually for 2 years, if stored in glass bottle and away from light, heat, security checks at airports, exposure to radiation.

COMMONLY ASKED QUESTIONS AND ANSWERS

Q. Can I take homeopathic medicines alongwith the allopathic medicines which I am already taking?

Ans. In certain situations, yes, while in other situations, these are inimical to each other.

Following few examples will illustrate this:

a) Hepar sulf will clash with antibiotics.

b) Allium cepa will clash with antihistamine (cetrizine, actifed, avil).

In other situations, where antibiotics are a must, their side-effects like gastric pain or diarrhoea of allopathic drugs can be counteracted with homeopathy.

In certain situations, both allopathic and homeopathic medicines can be given as complementary to each other until the time homeopathy takes control, then we can stop allopathic medicines. As an example, I have always adopted this procedure in patients who have been taking allopathic medicine for high blood pressure.

Again, it is very important to note that steroids clash with homeopathy. Giving homeopathic medicines in cases of steroids will aggravate their symptoms.

Conclusively, each case has to be judged on its own merits.

Q. Can a diabetic take these sweet homeopathic tablets?
Ans. In controlled and restricted amount of sweet pills (lactose or glucose), it can be taken. However, I often advise them to take in liquid form, which is safer, if the medication has to be taken for a longer period.

Q. Storage: Should it be in refrigerator or at ordinary temperature?
Ans. It should be at ordinary room temperature, but away from humidity, moisture and excessive heat.

Q. Any food restrictions?
Ans. It depends on the type of remedy in relation to food. For example:
a) Onions should be avoided with allium cepa.
b) There is no need of restriction of onions with other remedies.
c) Spicy food should be avoided with capsicum and nux vomica. Coffee should be avoided with coffea.

Q. Can radiation at security checks at airports affect the effect of the remedies?
Ans. According to my experience, no. I had taken with me and my patients homeopathic medicines abroad, and they have worked effectively despite going through security checks by radiation scanners. However, repeated exposure to radiations can affect the efficacy. To counteract the effect of security radiations, I have bought **lead** small bag, usually available in photographers' shops. The lead bag does protect from radiation to some extent.

Q. Can there be an allergic reaction to homeopathic medicines?
Ans. In certain situations, yes. The following examples will illustrate.

One of my patients, a renowned dermatologist, reacted badly and later on I discovered that she had lactose intolerance (sugar pills – the vehicle for homeopathy).

At times, I have noticed hypersensitivity reaction. If a patient shows good improvement to a particular remedy, next time he reacts badly to the same remedy unless you give it in higher potency than what was given previously.

Q. Any side-effects of mother tinctures?

Ans. The only unpleasant side-effects of mother tincture are increased acidity and gastric upset, even with those which are indicated for gastric problems. The reason behind this is the alcohol content of these mother tinctures. So, I often advise mother tinctures to be taken after meals or I give antacid pills alongwith these.